HOW TO STOP BINGE EATING

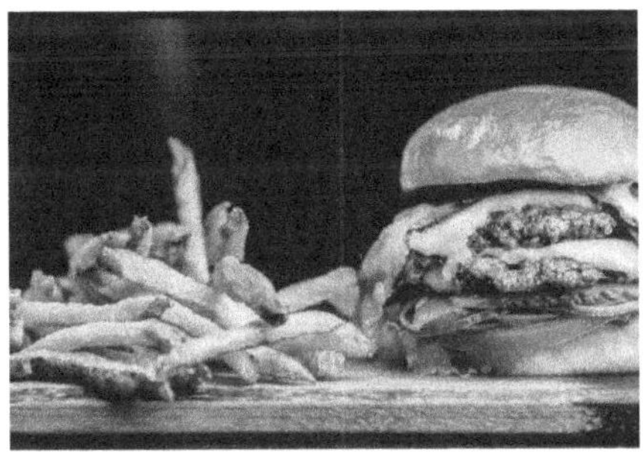

Strategies and Support for Overcoming Binge Eating"

EMMA LYNCH

TABLE OF CONTENTS

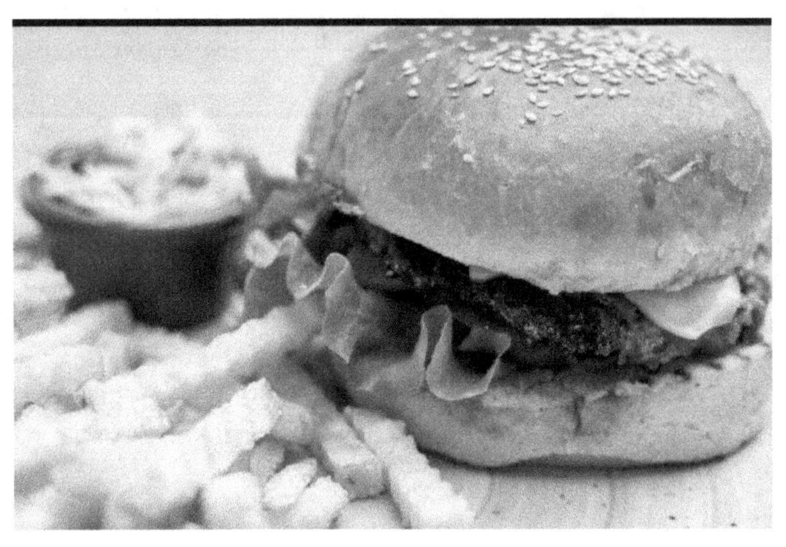

INTRODUCTION

Binge eating is a complex and often distressing behavior characterized by consuming large quantities of food in a short period, accompanied by a sense of loss of control. It can have profound effects on both physical and emotional well-being, leading to feelings of guilt, shame, and self-loathing. However, overcoming binge eating is possible with the right strategies and support.

Understanding binge eating is the first step toward recovery. It often stems from a combination of psychological, social, and biological factors. Emotional triggers, such as stress, anxiety, or depression, can lead individuals to turn to food as a coping mechanism. Additionally, societal pressures, diet culture, and negative body image can exacerbate binge eating behaviors.

Addressing binge eating requires a multifaceted approach. It involves recognizing triggers, developing healthy coping mechanisms, and building a support system. Mindful eating techniques can help individuals reconnect with their bodies and understand the difference between physical and emotional hunger. Developing a well-rounded meal plan that emphasizes providing the body with wholesome nutrients can also be very important in controlling binge eating.

Moreover, seeking professional help, whether through therapy, counseling, or support groups, can provide invaluable guidance and support on the journey to recovery. By addressing underlying issues and developing sustainable strategies, individuals can break free from the cycle of binge eating and reclaim their health and happiness. This guide will explore various techniques and resources to help individuals overcome binge eating and foster a positive relationship with food and their bodies.

CHAPTER ONE

UNDERSTANDING BINGE EATING

Binge eating is a multifaceted psychological disorder characterized by recurrent episodes of consuming unusually large amounts of food in a discrete period, often accompanied by a sense of loss of control. Unlike other eating disorders such as anorexia nervosa or bulimia nervosa, individuals with binge eating disorder (BED) do not engage in compensatory behaviors such as purging, fasting, or excessive exercise to counteract the effects of overeating. Instead, they experience intense feelings of guilt, shame, and distress following binge episodes.

To comprehend binge eating fully, it's crucial to explore its various dimensions:

1. Psychological Factors:

 - Emotional Triggers: Stress, anxiety, loneliness, and despair are typical emotional distressors that trigger binge eating. Food may be used as a coping mechanism to numb or alleviate uncomfortable emotions.

 - Negative Body Image: Individuals with binge eating disorder may have distorted perceptions of their bodies and engage in binge eating as a way to cope with negative body image or low self-esteem.

  - Dieting and Restriction: Paradoxically, attempts to control food intake through restrictive dieting can trigger binge eating episodes. Restriction leads to feelings of deprivation, which can increase the likelihood of overeating during binge episodes.

2. Social and Environmental Factors:

  - Diet Culture: Societal pressures to conform to unrealistic beauty standards and the prevalence of diet culture can contribute to the development of binge eating behaviors.

  - Family Dynamics: Dysfunctional family dynamics, such as chaotic or emotionally invalidating environments, may also play a role in the development of binge eating disorder.

3. Biological Factors:

  - Genetics: There is evidence to suggest that genetic factors play a role in the development of binge eating disorder. Individuals with a family history of eating disorders or mood disorders may be at a higher risk of developing binge eating behaviors.

  - Neurotransmitter Imbalances: Abnormalities in brain chemistry, particularly involving neurotransmitters such as serotonin and dopamine, may contribute to the dysregulation of appetite and impulse control seen in binge eating disorder.

Understanding binge eating involves recognizing the interplay between these psychological, social, and biological factors. It is not simply a matter of lacking willpower or self-control but rather a complex interaction of genetic, environmental, and psychological influences. By addressing these underlying factors through therapy, counseling, and behavioral interventions, individuals can begin to unravel the patterns of binge eating and work towards developing healthier coping mechanisms and a healthier connection between food and their bodies.

WHY IT'S IMPORTANT TO ADDRESS BINGE EATING

It's crucial to address binge eating for several reasons, as it can have significant impacts on both physical and psychological well-being:

1. Health Risks: Binge eating often involves consuming large quantities of high-calorie, low-nutrient foods, which can lead to weight gain, obesity, and related health conditions such as type 2 diabetes, high blood pressure, and heart disease. Chronic binge eating can also result in gastrointestinal issues, metabolic disturbances, and nutritional deficiencies.

2. Emotional Distress: Binge eating is accompanied by intense feelings of guilt, shame, and distress,

which can significantly impact an individual's mental health and quality of life. The cycle of bingeing and subsequent negative emotions can contribute to low self-esteem, depression, anxiety, and other mood disorders, further perpetuating the cycle of binge eating.

3. Social Isolation: Individuals struggling with binge eating may experience social withdrawal and isolation due to feelings of embarrassment or shame surrounding their eating behaviors. This can lead to strained relationships with friends and family, as well as feelings of loneliness and alienation.

4. Impaired Functioning: Binge eating can cause problems with day-to-day functioning, making it harder to accomplish tasks at work, school, or other commitments. The preoccupation with food and body image, as well as the physical discomfort and emotional distress associated with binge episodes, can make it challenging to focus, concentrate, or engage in activities of daily living.

5. Risk of Co-occurring Disorders: Binge eating often co-occurs with other mental health conditions, such as depression, anxiety, and substance abuse disorders. Addressing binge eating is essential to prevent the development or exacerbation of these co-occurring disorders and to promote overall well-being.

6. Long-term Health Outcomes: Untreated binge eating disorder is associated with a range of long-term health consequences, including increased risk of obesity-related comorbidities, decreased life expectancy, and reduced quality of life. Addressing binge eating early can help mitigate these risks and improve long-term health outcomes.

Overall, addressing binge eating is crucial for promoting physical health, emotional well-being, and overall quality of life. Seeking professional help and support can empower individuals to break free from the cycle of binge eating, develop healthier coping mechanisms, and cultivate a positive relationship with food and their bodies.

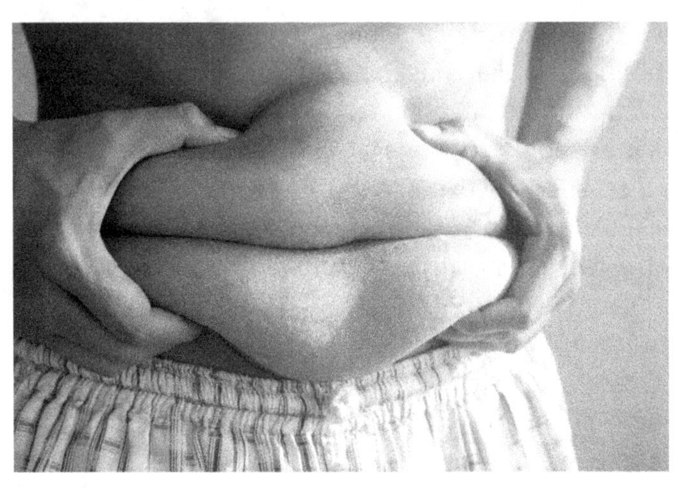

CHAPTER TWO

RECOGNIZING TRIGGERS

Finding triggers is a crucial initial step in treating binge eating disorder (BED) and regaining control over one's eating habits. The internal or environmental stimuli known as triggers cause or intensify episodes of binge eating. By identifying and understanding these triggers, individuals can develop strategies to manage them effectively. Triggers for binge eating can vary widely from person to person but commonly include:

1. Emotional Triggers:

- Stress: High levels of stress can lead to feelings of overwhelm, prompting individuals to turn to food as a coping mechanism.

- Anxiety: Feelings of anxiety or nervousness may trigger a desire to soothe oneself with food, leading to binge eating episodes.

- Depression: Low mood and feelings of sadness or hopelessness can prompt individuals to seek comfort in food to temporarily alleviate emotional pain.

2. Environmental Triggers:

- Food Availability: The presence of tempting or highly palatable foods in the environment can trigger cravings and lead to binge eating.

- Social Situations: Social gatherings, parties, or celebrations where food is abundant may trigger overeating in response to social pressure or emotional cues.

- Time of Day: Certain times of day, such as late at night or after a stressful day at work, may be more prone to triggering binge eating episodes.

3. Physiological Triggers:

- Hunger and Fullness: Disruptions in hunger and satiety cues, such as skipping meals or restrictive dieting, can lead to intense hunger and subsequent overeating.

- Hormonal Changes: Fluctuations in hormones, such as during menstruation or menopause, may influence appetite and trigger binge eating behaviors.

Recognizing triggers involves increased self-awareness and mindfulness of one's thoughts, feelings, and behaviors surrounding food and eating. Keeping a food and mood journal can be helpful in identifying patterns and associations between emotional states and binge eating episodes. Once triggers are identified, individuals can develop coping strategies to manage them effectively, such as practicing stress-reduction techniques, finding alternative ways to cope with emotions, and creating a supportive environment that promotes healthy eating habits. By addressing triggers proactively, individuals can reduce the frequency and severity of binge eating episodes and take steps towards recovery.

IDENTIFYING EMOTIONAL TRIGGERS

Identifying emotional triggers is crucial in understanding and managing binge eating behavior. Emotional triggers are internal cues that prompt individuals to turn to food as a coping mechanism to soothe or suppress difficult emotions. By recognizing these triggers, individuals can develop healthier ways of coping with emotions and reduce the likelihood of engaging in binge eating episodes. Here are some strategies for identifying emotional triggers:

1. Self-Reflection: Take time to reflect on your thoughts, feelings, and behaviors surrounding food and eating. Notice patterns and associations between specific emotions and binge eating episodes. Ask yourself questions such as:
   - What emotions am I experiencing before, during, and after a binge eating episode?
   - Are there particular situations or events that consistently trigger binge eating?
   - How do I feel physically and emotionally during a binge eating episode?

2. Keep a Food and Mood Journal: Start a journal to track your food intake, cravings, emotions, and

the circumstances surrounding binge eating episodes. Record details such as:
  - The time and location of the binge eating episode
  - The types of foods consumed
  - The emotions you were experiencing before and during the episode
  - Any specific triggers or stressors present at the time

3. Pay Attention to Physical Sensations: Notice how your body responds to different emotions. Emotional eating often involves a disconnect between physical hunger and emotional hunger. Before reaching for food, pause and ask yourself if you're truly hungry or if there might be an emotional need driving the desire to eat.

4. Identify Common Themes: Look for common themes or patterns among your emotional triggers. Are certain emotions, such as stress, loneliness, boredom, or sadness, more likely to trigger binge eating episodes? Are there specific situations or triggers, such as social gatherings, conflict, or deadlines, that consistently lead to overeating?

5. Seek Professional Support: Consider seeking guidance from a therapist, counselor, or registered dietitian with experience in treating binge eating disorder. They can help you explore underlying emotional triggers, develop coping strategies, and provide support on your journey to recovery.

By identifying emotional triggers for binge eating, individuals can gain insight into their eating behaviors and develop more adaptive ways of coping with difficult emotions. This self-awareness is a crucial step towards breaking the cycle of binge eating and fostering a healthier relationship with food and emotions.

RECOGNIZING ENVIRONMENTAL TRIGGERS

Recognizing environmental triggers is key for understanding and managing binge eating behavior. Environmental triggers are external cues or circumstances in the surroundings that can prompt individuals to engage in binge eating episodes. By identifying these triggers, individuals can make changes to their environment and develop strategies to cope more effectively. Here are some common environmental triggers and strategies for recognizing them:

1. Food Availability:
   - Recognize situations where tempting or highly palatable foods are readily accessible, such as at parties, social gatherings, or in the home.
   - Take note of environments where unhealthy foods are prevalent, such as at work, school, or in certain social circles.

- Pay attention to the presence of trigger foods—those foods that are particularly difficult to resist or control consumption of.

2. Social Situations:
- Identify social situations that may lead to overeating, such as dining out with friends, family gatherings, or celebrations.
- Notice how social pressure or peer influence may contribute to overeating in certain contexts.
- Be aware of emotional cues from others that may influence your eating behavior, such as comments about food or body image.

3. Time of Day:
- Notice if there are specific times of day when you are more prone to overeating, such as late at night or during periods of boredom.
- Pay attention to routines and habits that may influence eating patterns, such as snacking while watching TV or eating out of boredom during work breaks.

4. Emotional Atmosphere:
- Be mindful of the emotional atmosphere in your environment and how it may impact your eating behavior.
- Notice if stressful or chaotic environments contribute to feelings of anxiety or overwhelm, prompting a desire to turn to food for comfort.

- Identify environments that promote relaxation and mindfulness, which can help reduce the likelihood of engaging in emotional eating.

5. Triggers Outside the Home:
- Consider how external environments, such as restaurants, grocery stores, or advertisements, may influence your food choices and eating behaviors.
- Be aware of triggers related to food cues, such as seeing or smelling food, that may stimulate cravings or lead to overeating.

By recognizing environmental triggers for binge eating, individuals can take proactive steps to modify their surroundings and develop coping strategies to manage these triggers effectively. This may involve creating a supportive environment that promotes healthy eating habits, setting boundaries around food-related situations, and seeking support from friends, family, or healthcare professionals.

UNDERSTANDING PHYSIOLOGICAL TRIGGERS

Understanding physiological triggers is crucial for recognizing the internal cues that can prompt binge eating episodes. Physiological triggers are internal sensations or changes in the body that influence appetite, hunger, and eating behavior. By becoming aware of these physiological cues, individuals can develop strategies to manage them and reduce the likelihood of engaging in binge eating. Here are some common physiological triggers and strategies for understanding them:

1. Hunger and Satiety Cues:
   - Recognize the difference between physical hunger, which is a biological need for food, and emotional hunger, which is driven by psychological factors.
   - Pay attention to physical sensations such as stomach growling, lightheadedness, or weakness, which may indicate true hunger.
   - Notice how hunger and fullness levels fluctuate throughout the day and how they influence your eating behavior.

2. Blood Sugar Levels:
   - Understand how fluctuations in blood sugar levels can impact appetite and cravings.
   - Notice if feelings of low energy or fatigue coincide with cravings for sugary or high-carbohydrate foods.
   - Aim to stabilize blood sugar levels by consuming balanced meals and snacks that include protein, healthy fats, and fiber.

3. Hormonal Changes:
   - Be aware of how hormonal fluctuations, such as those related to the menstrual cycle, pregnancy, or menopause, may influence appetite and eating behavior.

- Notice if cravings for certain foods intensify during specific phases of the menstrual cycle or hormonal changes.
- Consider strategies for managing hormonal fluctuations, such as practicing stress reduction techniques, getting regular exercise, and maintaining a balanced diet.

4. Emotional Regulation:

- Understand the connection between emotions and physiological responses in the body, such as the release of stress hormones like cortisol.
- Notice if physiological sensations, such as tension or discomfort, coincide with emotional triggers for binge eating.
- Develop strategies for regulating emotions and managing stress in healthy ways, such as through mindfulness, deep breathing exercises, or physical activity.

5. Sleep and Fatigue:

- Recognize how lack of sleep or fatigue can impact appetite regulation and food cravings.
- Notice if feelings of tiredness or exhaustion lead to increased cravings for high-calorie, energy-dense foods.
- Prioritize adequate sleep and rest to support overall well-being and reduce the risk of binge eating triggered by fatigue.

By understanding physiological triggers for binge eating, individuals can develop greater self-awareness and make informed choices about their eating behavior. This may involve tuning into bodily cues, practicing mindful eating, and adopting healthy lifestyle habits that support overall well-being. Additionally, seeking support from healthcare professionals or therapists can provide valuable guidance and assistance in managing physiological triggers and promoting a balanced relationship with food.

CHAPTER THREE

MINDFUL EATING TECHNIQUES

Mindful eating techniques involve paying attention to the present moment and being fully aware of your eating experience without judgment. These practices can help individuals develop a healthier relationship with food, tune into their body's hunger and satiety cues, and reduce the likelihood of engaging in binge eating behaviors. Here are some mindful eating techniques to consider:

1. Eat without Distractions:

- Minimize distractions such as television, phones, or computers while eating.
- Focus solely on the sensory experience of eating, including the taste, texture, aroma, and temperature of the food.

2. Engage Your Senses:

- Before taking a bite, take a moment to observe the appearance of the food on your plate.
- Notice the smell of the food and how it activates your appetite.
- Take small bites and chew slowly, paying attention to the flavors and textures as you eat.

3. Listen to Your Body:

- Tune into your body's hunger and fullness cues before, during, and after eating.

- Consider whether you're eating because of habit, boredom, or emotional reasons rather than whether you're actually hungry.

- Stop eating when you feel satisfied, rather than waiting until you feel overly full.

4. Practice Non-Judgment:

- Eat with an open mind and curiosity, and refrain from categorizing food as "good" or "bad."

- Notice any judgments or criticisms that arise about your eating habits or food choices and let them go.

- Cultivate self-compassion and kindness toward yourself, recognizing that everyone has unique preferences and needs.

5. Cultivate Gratitude:

- Take a moment to express gratitude for the food you're about to eat and the nourishment it provides to your body.

- Reflect on the journey of the food from farm to table and the effort that went into producing it.

- Appreciate the opportunity to savor and enjoy each bite of food, rather than rushing through the eating process.

6. Mindful Eating Exercises:

- Practice mindful eating exercises, such as the raisin exercise or mindful eating meditation, to deepen your awareness of eating habits and sensations.

- Experiment with incorporating mindfulness practices into mealtime rituals, such as taking a few deep breaths before eating or saying a silent blessing or affirmation.

By incorporating mindful eating techniques into your daily routine, you can cultivate a more balanced and attuned relationship with food. These practices can help you become more aware of your eating habits, recognize triggers for binge eating, and develop healthier coping mechanisms for managing emotions and stress. Over time, mindful eating can lead to greater satisfaction, enjoyment, and peace around food and eating.

PRACTICING MINDFUL EATING

Practicing mindful eating involves bringing full attention and awareness to the experience of eating, without judgment or distraction. It's about being present in the moment and tuning into your body's hunger and satiety cues, as well as the sensory experience of eating. Here's how to practice mindful eating:

1. **Start with Intention**: Begin your meal with a moment of intention or gratitude. Take a few deep breaths to center yourself and express gratitude for the nourishment the food provides.

2. **Engage Your Senses**: Before taking a bite, take a moment to observe the appearance of the food on your plate. Notice the colors, shapes, and textures. Smell the aroma of the food and how it stimulates your appetite.

3. **Eat Slowly and Chew Thoroughly**: Take small bites and chew your food slowly and thoroughly. Pay attention to the taste, texture, and sensations of each bite as you chew.

4. **Pause Between Bites**: After swallowing a bite, pause for a moment before taking another. Notice any lingering flavors or sensations in your mouth. Check in with your body to see if you're still hungry or if you're starting to feel satisfied.

5. **Tune into Hunger and Fullness**: Throughout the meal, check in with your body to assess your hunger and fullness levels. Notice the physical sensations of hunger in your stomach and the feeling of satisfaction as you eat.

6. **Notice Emotional Triggers**: Pay attention to any emotional cues or triggers that arise during the meal. Observe if you're eating because you're bored, stressed, or experiencing other feelings. Practice observing these emotions without judgment or the need to act on them.

7. **Minimize Distractions**: Eat without distractions such as television, phones, or

computers. Focus solely on the experience of eating and the sensations in your body.

8. **Practice Gratitude**: Express gratitude for the food you're eating and the nourishment it provides to your body. Reflect on the journey of the food from farm to table and the effort that went into producing it.

9. **Listen to Your Body**: Pay attention to your body's signals of hunger and fullness. Stop eating when you feel satisfied, rather than waiting until you feel overly full. Trust your body to guide you in knowing when you've had enough.

10. **Reflect on the Experience**: After finishing your meal, take a moment to reflect on the experience of eating mindfully. Notice any changes in how you feel physically, mentally, or emotionally. Consider how practicing mindful eating can benefit your overall well-being.

By practicing mindful eating regularly, you can develop a deeper connection to your body's needs, cultivate a more positive relationship with food, and reduce the likelihood of engaging in binge eating behaviors.

UNDERSTANDING HUNGER CUES

Understanding hunger cues is essential for practicing mindful eating and developing a healthy relationship with food. Hunger cues are the body's signals indicating the need for nourishment and energy. By tuning into these cues, individuals can learn to distinguish between physical hunger and other factors that may influence eating behaviors, such as emotions or external cues. Here's how to understand hunger cues:

1. **Physical Sensations**: Pay attention to physical sensations in your body that indicate hunger, such as stomach growling, feelings of emptiness or gnawing in the stomach, or a slight headache. These sensations are signs that your body needs fuel to function optimally.

2. **Timing**: Notice the timing of your meals and snacks throughout the day. Regularly spaced meals and snacks help maintain stable blood sugar levels and prevent extreme hunger or overeating later in the day.

3. **Gradual Onset**: True physical hunger typically develops gradually over time and increases in intensity if not satisfied. It may start as a mild sensation and gradually become more noticeable over the course of several hours.

4. **Specific Cravings**: Pay attention to specific cravings or desires for certain foods. True hunger is usually open to a variety of food options, while cravings driven by emotions or external cues may be more specific or intense.

5. **Energy Levels**: Notice how your energy levels fluctuate throughout the day. True physical hunger is often accompanied by feelings of fatigue or weakness, indicating the body's need for fuel.

6. **Emotional State**: Consider your emotional state and how it may influence your perception of hunger. Emotional hunger is typically sudden and intense, triggered by emotions such as stress, boredom, or sadness, rather than physical sensations in the body.

7. **External Cues**: Be aware of external cues that may influence your eating behavior, such as the sight or smell of food, social situations, or the time of day. These cues can sometimes override true physical hunger signals and lead to mindless or emotional eating.

8. **Thirst**: Recognize the difference between hunger and thirst. Sometimes, feelings of hunger may actually be a sign of dehydration. Drink a glass of water and wait a few minutes to see if the hunger subsides before reaching for food.

9. **Mind-Body Connection**: Develop greater awareness of the mind-body connection and how your thoughts, emotions, and physical sensations interact. Notice how your thoughts and emotions may influence your perception of hunger and eating behavior.

10. **Hunger vs. Appetite**: Distinguish between hunger, which is a physical need for food, and appetite, which is the desire to eat for pleasure or enjoyment. Learn to honor your body's hunger cues while also being mindful of your appetite and preferences.

By understanding hunger cues and learning to listen to your body's signals, you can make more informed choices about when, what, and how much to eat. Practicing mindful eating techniques can help you develop a deeper connection to your body's needs and promote a healthier relationship with food.

LEARNING TO DIFFERENTIATE BETWEEN PHYSICAL AND EMOTIONAL HUNGER

Learning to differentiate between physical and emotional hunger is a crucial aspect of mindful eating and developing a healthy relationship with food. While physical hunger is driven by the body's need for nourishment and energy, emotional hunger is often triggered by psychological factors such as stress, boredom, or sadness. The following techniques can be used to help distinguish between the two:

1. **Physical Hunger**:
   - Develops gradually over time.
   - Accompanied by physical sensations such as stomach growling, feelings of emptiness or gnawing in the stomach, or a slight headache.
   - Open to a variety of food options and satisfied by nourishing, balanced meals and snacks.
   - Typically occurs in response to the body's physiological need for fuel and energy to function optimally.
   - Subsides once the body's energy needs are met and is typically associated with feelings of satisfaction and fullness.

2. **Emotional Hunger**:
   - Often sudden and intense, triggered by emotions such as stress, boredom, loneliness, or sadness.
   - Cravings are often specific and targeted towards comfort foods high in sugar, fat, or carbohydrates.
   - Not typically relieved by eating, as the underlying emotional needs are not addressed.
   - May be accompanied by feelings of guilt, shame, or regret after eating, especially if the food choices were made impulsively or mindlessly.
   - can cause mental anguish and recurrent behaviors of overeating if left untreated.

**Strategies for Differentiating Between Physical
and Emotional Hunger:**

1. **Check In with Yourself**: Take a moment to
evaluate your level of hunger before reaching for
any food. Ask yourself if you're truly physically
hungry or if there may be other factors at play, such
as emotions or external cues.

2. **Identify Triggers**: Notice any emotional
triggers or cues that may prompt feelings of hunger.
Pay attention to situations, events, or emotions that
tend to trigger cravings or the desire to eat.

3. **Mindfulness Practices**: Practice
mindfulness techniques to bring awareness to your
thoughts, emotions, and physical sensations in the
present moment. Notice any patterns or
associations between emotions and eating
behaviors.

4. **Emotional Awareness**: Develop greater
emotional awareness and learn to recognize and
name your emotions. Instead of turning to food to
cope with difficult emotions, explore alternative
coping strategies such as journaling, talking to a
friend, or engaging in a favorite hobby.

5. **Distraction Techniques**: If you suspect that
your hunger may be driven by emotions rather than
physical need, try engaging in a distracting activity

for a few minutes to see if the desire to eat subsides. Take a walk, listen to music, or practice deep breathing exercises to shift your focus away from food.

6. **Seek Support**: Reach out to friends, family, or a therapist for support if you're struggling with emotional eating. Talking to someone can help you process your emotions and develop healthier coping mechanisms for managing stress and difficult feelings.

By learning to differentiate between physical and emotional hunger, you can develop greater awareness of your eating habits and make more mindful choices about when, what, and how much to eat. This can help reduce the likelihood of engaging in emotional eating and promote a healthier relationship with food and your body.

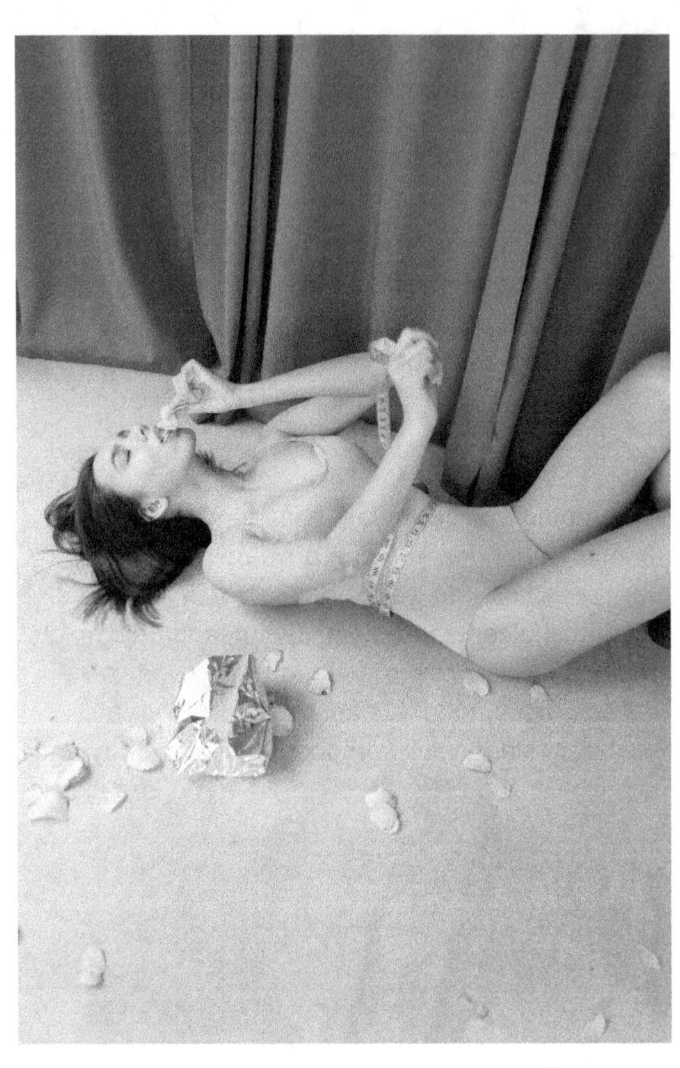

CHAPTER FOUR

BUILDING A SUPPORT SYSTEM

Building a support system is essential for individuals seeking to overcome binge eating disorder (BED) or develop a healthier relationship with food. A strong support network provides encouragement, guidance, and accountability, helping individuals navigate challenges and stay on track with their recovery journey. The following actions can assist in creating a support system:

1. **Identify Supportive Individuals**: Reach out to friends, family members, or trusted loved ones who can offer support and understanding. These individuals can serve as allies in your recovery journey, providing encouragement, empathy, and practical assistance when needed.

2. **Communicate Your Needs**: Be open and honest about your struggles with binge eating and your goals for recovery. Clearly communicate your needs and boundaries to your support system, and let them know how they can best support you on your journey.

3. **Seek Professional Help**: Consider seeking guidance from healthcare professionals, such as therapists, counselors, or registered dietitians, who specialize in treating BED or eating disorders.

These professionals can offer expert guidance, personalized treatment plans, and specialized interventions to support your recovery.

4. **Join Support Groups**: Look for support groups or online communities specifically for individuals struggling with binge eating or disordered eating. Connecting with others who are going through similar experiences can provide validation, empathy, and practical tips for managing challenges.

5. **Attend Therapy Sessions**: Participate in individual or group therapy sessions focused on addressing binge eating behaviors and underlying emotional issues. Therapy can help you explore the root causes of your binge eating, develop coping strategies, and build resilience in managing triggers.

6. **Engage in Peer Support**: Connect with peers who are also on a journey of recovery from binge eating or eating disorders. Peer support can offer a sense of camaraderie, shared understanding, and mutual encouragement in overcoming challenges and celebrating successes.

7. **Educate Your Support System**: Help educate your support system about binge eating disorder and how they can best support you in your recovery. Provide resources, information, and insights into the nature of BED, as well as

strategies for supporting someone with an eating disorder.

8. **Practice Self-Care**: Prioritize self-care activities that promote physical, emotional, and mental well-being. Engage in activities such as exercise, mindfulness practices, hobbies, and relaxation techniques to recharge and nourish yourself.

9. **Stay Connected**: Stay connected with your support system regularly, whether through phone calls, text messages, or in-person meetings. Check in with each other, share updates on your progress, and lean on each other for encouragement during challenging times.

10. **Express Gratitude**: Show appreciation for the support and encouragement you receive from your support system. Express gratitude for their presence in your life and the positive impact they have on your recovery journey.

By building a supportive network of individuals who understand and empathize with your struggles, you can feel less alone in your recovery journey and gain the strength and resilience needed to overcome binge eating disorder. Remember that recovery is a journey, and having a strong support system can make all the difference in achieving long-term success and well-being.

SEEKING PROFESSIONAL HELP

A vital first step in treating binge eating disorder (BED) and starting the healing process is getting expert assistance. Healthcare professionals, such as therapists, counselors, registered dietitians, and physicians, can provide expert guidance, personalized treatment plans, and specialized interventions to support individuals in their journey towards healing. The following justifies the significance of obtaining expert assistance:

1. **Expertise and Specialization**: Healthcare professionals who specialize in eating disorders have the knowledge, training, and experience to understand the complexities of BED and provide evidence-based treatment options tailored to individual needs.

2. **Comprehensive Assessment**: A thorough assessment by a healthcare professional can help determine the severity of binge eating behaviors, identify underlying factors contributing to BED, and evaluate any co-occurring mental health conditions or medical concerns that may need to be addressed.

3. **Personalized Treatment Plan**: Based on the assessment, healthcare professionals can develop a personalized treatment plan that addresses the unique needs, goals, and preferences of the individual. Treatment may include therapy,

nutritional counseling, medication management, and other interventions tailored to the individual's specific situation.

4. **Therapy and Counseling**: Therapy, such as cognitive-behavioral therapy (CBT) or dialectical behavior therapy (DBT), is often recommended as a first-line treatment for BED. Therapy can help individuals explore the underlying factors contributing to binge eating, develop coping strategies, challenge negative thoughts and beliefs about food and body image, and learn healthier ways of managing emotions and stress.

5. **Nutritional Counseling**: Registered dietitians specializing in eating disorders can provide guidance on developing a balanced and nourishing meal plan, navigating food-related challenges, and fostering a healthier relationship with food. Nutritional counseling can also address any dietary restrictions, food allergies, or medical conditions that may impact eating habits.

6. **Medication Management**: In some cases, healthcare professionals may prescribe medications, such as antidepressants or anti-anxiety medications, to help manage symptoms of BED and co-occurring mental health conditions. Medication management should be closely monitored by a qualified healthcare provider.

7. **Ongoing Support and Monitoring:**
Healthcare professionals provide ongoing support,
guidance, and monitoring throughout the recovery
process. Regular therapy sessions, check-ins, and
follow-up appointments allow for adjustments to
treatment plans as needed and help individuals
stay on track with their recovery goals.

8. **Collaborative Care:** Healthcare
professionals often work collaboratively as part of a
multidisciplinary team to provide holistic and
comprehensive care for individuals with BED.
Collaboration may involve communication and
coordination between therapists, dietitians,
physicians, and other healthcare providers to
ensure continuity of care and address all aspects of
the individual's well-being.

9. **Education and Resources:** Healthcare
professionals can provide education and resources
to help individuals and their families better
understand binge eating disorder, develop skills for
managing symptoms, and navigate challenges
related to recovery. Education empowers
individuals to make informed decisions about their
health and recovery journey.

10. **Hope and Encouragement:** Seeking
professional help offers individuals hope for
recovery and reassurance that they are not alone in
their struggles. Healthcare professionals provide
support, encouragement, and validation, helping

individuals feel understood, accepted, and empowered to overcome BED and reclaim their lives.

Overall, seeking professional help is a critical step towards healing from binge eating disorder and building a healthier relationship with food and body image. It's important to reach out for support and guidance from qualified professionals who can provide the care and resources needed to support recovery and promote overall well-being.

COMMUNICATING WITH FRIENDS AND FAMILY

Communicating with friends and family about binge eating disorder (BED) can be challenging but is essential for receiving support and understanding during the recovery process. Here are some tips for effectively communicating with loved ones about BED:

1. **Choose the Right Time and Place**: Find a private and comfortable setting to have open and honest conversations about BED. Choose a time when both you and your loved ones are calm and free from distractions.

2. **Be Honest and Open**: Approach the conversation with honesty and openness about your struggles with BED. Share your feelings,

experiences, and concerns with your loved ones, and be willing to listen to their perspectives as well.

3. **Educate Them About BED**: Provide information and resources to help your friends and family better understand binge eating disorder. Explain that BED is a recognized medical condition characterized by recurrent episodes of binge eating and is not simply a lack of willpower or self-control.

4. **Express Your Needs**: Clearly communicate your needs and boundaries to your friends and family. Let them know how they can best support you in your recovery journey, whether it's offering encouragement, providing accountability, or helping create a supportive environment.

5. **Set Realistic Expectations**: Help your loved ones understand that recovery from BED is a process that takes time, patience, and effort. Set realistic expectations for yourself and your loved ones, and emphasize that setbacks and challenges are a normal part of the journey.

6. **Encourage Open Dialogue**: Encourage open dialogue and communication with your friends and family about BED. Let them know that you're open to answering questions, addressing concerns, and discussing any challenges or successes along the way.

7. **Emphasize the Importance of Support:**
Stress the importance of having a supportive
network of friends and family members during the
recovery process. Let your loved ones know that
their support, encouragement, and understanding
play a crucial role in your healing and well-being.

8. **Seek Professional Help Together:** Consider
involving your friends and family in the recovery
process by attending therapy sessions or support
groups together. This can help foster a deeper
understanding of BED and provide opportunities for
shared learning and growth.

9. **Address Misconceptions and Stigma:** Be
prepared to address any misconceptions or stigma
surrounding binge eating disorder. Educate your
friends and family about the realities of BED and
challenge any harmful stereotypes or beliefs.

10. **Express Gratitude:** Show appreciation for
the support and understanding you receive from
your friends and family. Express gratitude for their
willingness to listen, learn, and be there for you
during your recovery journey.

By communicating openly and honestly with your
friends and family about binge eating disorder, you
can foster understanding, receive support, and
strengthen your relationships as you work towards
healing and recovery. Remind yourself that there

are people out there who genuinely care about you and want to see you succeed. You are not alone.

JOINING SUPPORT GROUP OR THERAPY SESSION

Joining a support group or therapy session can be immensely beneficial for individuals struggling with binge eating disorder (BED). Both options provide a supportive environment, opportunities for education and skill-building, and connections with others who understand your experiences. Here are some considerations for joining a support group or therapy session:

1. **Support Groups:**
  - Support groups bring together individuals who are facing similar challenges with BED, providing a sense of community, validation, and mutual support.
  - Support groups may be facilitated by healthcare professionals or peers with lived experience, offering different perspectives and insights into recovery.
  - Participating in a support group can help reduce feelings of isolation, shame, and stigma associated with BED, as well as provide opportunities for shared learning and growth.
  - Support groups may meet in person, online, or via phone, allowing for flexibility and accessibility based on individual preferences and needs.

- Think about joining a support group connected to trustworthy institutions like your neighborhood eating disorder treatment facilities or the National Eating Disorders Association (NEDA).

2. **Therapy Sessions**:
   - Therapy, such as cognitive-behavioral therapy (CBT), dialectical behavior therapy (DBT), or interpersonal therapy (IPT), is often recommended as a primary treatment for BED.
   - Therapy sessions provide a safe and confidential space to explore the underlying factors contributing to BED, develop coping strategies, challenge negative thoughts and behaviors, and build skills for managing emotions and stress.
   - Individual therapy allows for personalized treatment plans tailored to your specific needs, goals, and concerns related to BED.
   - Group therapy sessions may also be available, offering opportunities for peer support, feedback, and accountability in a structured therapeutic setting.
   - Consider seeking therapy from a licensed mental health professional with experience and expertise in treating eating disorders, who can provide specialized care and support throughout your recovery journey.

Factors to Consider When Choosing Between Support Groups and Therapy Sessions:

1. **Personal Preferences**: Consider your preferences for group dynamics, format (in-person, online, or phone), and level of structure when deciding between support groups and therapy sessions.

2. **Treatment Goals**: Assess your treatment goals and needs related to BED. If you're seeking structured treatment, skill-building, and individualized support, therapy sessions may be more suitable. If you're looking for peer support, validation, and shared experiences, a support group may be a better fit.

3. **Level of Care**: Consider the level of care needed based on the severity of your BED symptoms, co-occurring mental health conditions, and any previous treatment experiences. Therapy sessions may offer more intensive and focused treatment, while support groups provide ongoing support and connection.

4. **Accessibility and Availability**: Evaluate the accessibility and availability of support groups and therapy sessions in your area. Online options may be more accessible for individuals with limited transportation or scheduling conflicts.

5. **Combination Approach**: Some individuals benefit from a combination of support groups and therapy sessions, integrating different forms of support and treatment into their recovery plan.

Explore what combination of resources works best for you and your needs.

Ultimately, whether you choose to join a support group, therapy session, or both, seeking support and professional guidance is an important step towards healing from binge eating disorder. Remember that recovery is a journey, and having a supportive network and access to specialized treatment can make a significant difference in your path towards healing and well-being.

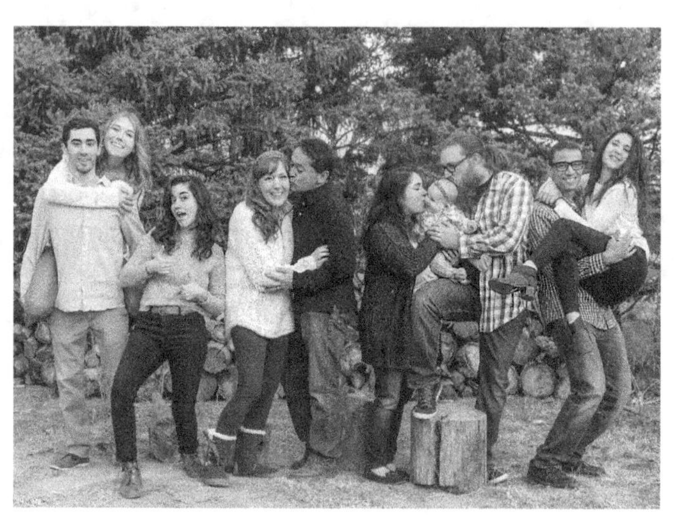

CHAPTER FIVE

DEVELOPING HEALTHY COPING MECHANISM

Developing healthy coping mechanisms is essential for individuals struggling with binge eating disorder (BED) to manage emotions, reduce stress, and maintain a balanced relationship with food. In addition to addressing the underlying causes of binge eating, healthy coping techniques can help people become more resilient and enhance their general wellbeing. Here are some effective coping mechanisms for managing BED:

1. **Mindfulness and Meditation**:
   - Practice mindfulness techniques, such as deep breathing exercises, meditation, or yoga, to cultivate awareness of thoughts, emotions, and bodily sensations in the present moment.
   - Mindfulness can help individuals develop a non-judgmental and accepting attitude towards their experiences, reducing impulsivity and emotional reactivity that may contribute to binge eating.

2. **Emotion Regulation Skills**:
   - Learn emotion regulation skills to identify, understand, and manage difficult emotions in healthy ways.

- Use coping strategies such as journaling, expressive arts, or talking to a trusted friend or therapist to process and express emotions effectively.

3. **Stress Management Techniques**:
   - Practice stress management techniques such as progressive muscle relaxation, guided imagery, or aromatherapy to reduce feelings of tension and anxiety.
   - Engage in activities that promote relaxation and self-care, such as taking a warm bath, spending time in nature, or listening to calming music.

4. **Healthy Distractions**:
   - Take part in activities that make you feel good or fulfilled while diverting your attention from cravings for binge eating.
   - Find hobbies or interests that are enjoyable and engaging, such as reading, gardening, painting, or playing a musical instrument.

5. **Physical Activity**:
   - Incorporate regular physical activity into your routine to boost mood, reduce stress, and improve overall well-being.
   - Choose activities that you enjoy and can sustain long-term, such as walking, swimming, dancing, or yoga.

6. **Nutritional Self-Care**:

- Focus on nourishing your body with balanced and satisfying meals and snacks throughout the day.
- Prioritize regular mealtimes and include a variety of nutrient-rich foods such as fruits, vegetables, whole grains, lean proteins, and healthy fats.

7. **Self-Compassion and Self-Care**:
- Practice self-compassion and kindness towards yourself, recognizing that setbacks and challenges are a normal part of the recovery process.
- Prioritize self-care activities that nurture your physical, emotional, and mental well-being, such as getting adequate sleep, setting boundaries, and engaging in activities that bring joy and fulfillment.

8. **Social Support**:
- Consult with friends, family, or support groups for assistance; they may provide understanding, encouragement, and empathy.
- Stay connected with supportive individuals who validate your experiences and provide a sense of belonging and connection.

9. **Cognitive Restructuring**:
- Challenge negative thoughts and beliefs about food, body image, and self-worth through cognitive restructuring techniques.
- Replace negative self-talk with more balanced and compassionate perspectives that promote self-acceptance and resilience.

10. **Professional Help**:
   - Consider seeking guidance from healthcare professionals, such as therapists, counselors, or registered dietitians, who specialize in treating BED. Professional support can provide additional coping strategies, personalized treatment plans, and accountability in your recovery journey.

By incorporating healthy coping mechanisms into your daily life, individuals can develop resilience, manage emotions effectively, and reduce the frequency and intensity of binge eating episodes. Remember that building new coping skills takes time and practice, so be patient with yourself and celebrate progress along the way.

FINDING ALTERNATIVE WAYS TO COPE WITH STRESS

Finding alternative ways to cope with stress is essential for individuals struggling with binge eating disorder (BED) to reduce reliance on food as a coping mechanism and develop healthier habits for managing emotions. Here are some alternative strategies for coping with stress:

1. **Physical Activity**:
   - Engage in regular physical activity to release endorphins and reduce feelings of stress and tension.

- Choose activities that you enjoy, such as walking, jogging, cycling, dancing, or practicing yoga, and aim for at least 30 minutes of exercise most days of the week.

2. **Mindfulness and Relaxation Techniques**:

- Practice mindfulness meditation, deep breathing exercises, or progressive muscle relaxation to calm the mind and body and reduce stress.
- Set aside a few minutes each day to practice mindfulness or relaxation techniques, either on your own or using guided meditation apps or videos.

3. **Creative Expression**:

- Express yourself creatively through activities such as painting, drawing, writing, or playing music.
- Engaging in creative expression can provide a sense of catharsis, self-expression, and emotional release, helping to alleviate stress and promote well-being.

4. **Social Support**:

- Reach out to friends, family members, or support groups for emotional support and connection during times of stress.
- Share your feelings and experiences with trusted individuals who can offer empathy, encouragement, and validation.

5. **Healthy Distractions**:

- Find healthy distractions to occupy your mind and redirect your focus away from stressors.

- Engage in activities that bring you joy and fulfillment, such as reading, watching a movie, gardening, cooking, or spending time with pets.

6. **Journaling**:

- Keep a journal to express your thoughts, feelings, and experiences in writing.
- Use journaling as a tool for self-reflection, problem-solving, and emotional processing, helping to gain clarity and perspective on stressful situations.

7. **Self-Care Activities**:

- Prioritize self-care activities that promote your physical, emotional, and mental health.
- Take time for activities that promote relaxation and rejuvenation, such as taking a warm bath, practicing skincare routines, or indulging in hobbies you enjoy.

8. **Healthy Eating Habits**:

- Focus on nourishing your body with balanced and satisfying meals and snacks throughout the day.
- Choose nutrient-rich foods that provide sustained energy and support overall well-being, rather than turning to highly processed or sugary foods as a coping mechanism.

9. **Limiting Exposure to Stressors**:

- Identify and minimize exposure to sources of stress whenever possible, whether they're related to work, relationships, or other areas of life.
  - Set boundaries, prioritize tasks, and delegate responsibilities to reduce feelings of overwhelm and prevent stress from accumulating.

10. **Seeking Professional Help:**
  - If stress becomes overwhelming or unmanageable, consider seeking guidance from a therapist, counselor, or healthcare professional who can provide additional support, coping strategies, and resources.

By incorporating alternative coping strategies into your daily routine, individuals can reduce reliance on food as a coping mechanism and develop healthier habits for managing stress. Experiment with different techniques to find what works best for you and remember to be patient and compassionate with yourself as you navigate the journey towards healthier coping mechanisms.

ENGAGING IN HOBBIES AND ACTIVITIES

Engaging in hobbies and activities is a wonderful way to cope with stress, distract from urges to binge eat, and cultivate a sense of fulfillment and joy in life. Here are some ideas for hobbies and activities to explore:

1. **Creative Pursuits**:
   - Painting, drawing, sketching, or coloring
   - Writing poetry, stories, or journaling
   - Crafting, such as knitting, crocheting, or sewing
   - Photography or scrapbooking
   - Playing a musical instrument or singing

2. **Outdoor Activities**:
   - Jogging, walking, or hiking in the outdoors
   - Gardening or tending to indoor plants
   - Birdwatching or nature photography
   - Cycling or rollerblading in local parks or trails
   - Picnicking or having a leisurely outdoor meal

3. **Mind-Body Practices**:
   - Yoga or tai chi
   - Pilates or barre workouts
   - Meditation or mindfulness exercises
   - Guided relaxation or visualization techniques
   - Dance or movement therapy classes

4. **Learning and Skill-Building**:
   - Taking classes or workshops in subjects of interest
   - Learning a new language or musical instrument
   - Cooking or baking new recipes
   - DIY home improvement projects or renovations
   - Studying topics related to personal or professional development

5. **Community Involvement**:

- Volunteering for local charities or organizations
- Participating in community clean-up events or fundraisers
- Joining clubs or groups based on shared interests (e.g., book clubs, hiking groups, crafting circles)
- Attending cultural events, art exhibits, or performances in your area

6. **Physical Activities**:
- Joining recreational sports leagues or fitness classes
- Playing team sports such as soccer, basketball, or volleyball
- Swimming, surfing, or paddleboarding
- Rock climbing or indoor bouldering
- Trying adventurous activities like zip-lining, kayaking, or stand-up paddleboarding

7. **Culinary Exploration**:
- Trying new recipes or experimenting with different cuisines
- Visiting specialty food stores or farmers' markets
- Putting together meals for loved ones or throwing dinner parties
- Taking cooking or baking classes
- Starting a food blog or Instagram account to share your culinary creations

8. **Socializing and Connecting**:
- enjoying time with friends and family

- Organizing game nights, movie marathons, or potluck dinners
- Attending social events, parties, or gatherings in your community
- Joining online forums or social media groups related to your hobbies and interests
- Participating in virtual meetups or video calls with friends and family members

Engaging in hobbies and activities that bring you joy, fulfillment, and a sense of accomplishment can be a powerful way to cope with stress and promote overall well-being. Experiment with different activities, explore new interests, and prioritize self-care by making time for hobbies that nourish your mind, body, and soul.

LEARNING RELAXATION TECHNIQUES

Learning relaxation techniques can be incredibly beneficial for managing stress, reducing anxiety, and promoting overall well-being. Consider attempting these relaxing methods:

1. **Deep Breathing**:
- Find a comfortable position, either sitting or lying down.
- Close your eyes and take a deep breath in through your nose, allowing your belly to rise as you inhale.

- Hold your breath for a moment, then exhale slowly through your mouth, allowing your belly to fall.
- Continue breathing deeply and slowly, focusing on the sensation of the breath as it enters and leaves your body.

2. **Progressive Muscle Relaxation (PMR)**:

- Start by tensing the muscles in your toes and feet as tightly as you can for a few seconds.
- Then, release the tension and allow the muscles to relax completely, noticing the difference between tension and relaxation.
- Gradually work your way up through the rest of your body, tensing and relaxing each muscle group, including your calves, thighs, buttocks, abdomen, chest, arms, shoulders, neck, and face.
- Before going on to the next muscle group, give each one enough time to completely relax.

3. **Guided Imagery**:

- Close your eyes and imagine yourself in a peaceful and serene place, such as a beach, forest, or mountaintop.
- Use all of your senses to vividly imagine the sights, sounds, smells, and sensations of being in this peaceful place.
- Focus on your breathing as you immerse yourself in the imagery, allowing yourself to feel calm and relaxed.

4. **Mindfulness Meditation**:

- Find a comfortable position and bring your attention to your breath, noticing the sensation of the breath as it enters and leaves your body.
   - As thoughts or distractions arise, simply acknowledge them without judgment and gently bring your focus back to your breath.
   - Practice being fully present in the moment, observing your thoughts, emotions, and bodily sensations with curiosity and acceptance.

5. **Body Scan Meditation**:
   - Assume a comfortable laying position and focus on your body.
   - Starting from your toes, slowly scan your body from head to toe, noticing any areas of tension, discomfort, or relaxation.
   - With each breath, consciously release any tension or tightness you may be holding in your body, allowing yourself to sink deeper into a state of relaxation.

6. **Visualization**:
   - Imagine yourself in a peaceful and calming scene, such as a meadow, garden, or mountain retreat.
   - Picture yourself surrounded by beauty, tranquility, and serenity, and allow yourself to experience a sense of calm and relaxation as you immerse yourself in the visualization.

7. **Breath Counting**:

- Shut your eyes while you sit or lie down in a comfortable position.
- Take a deep breath in through your nose and count silently to yourself as you inhale.
- Then, exhale slowly through your mouth, counting silently to yourself again as you exhale.
- Continue this pattern, counting each inhale and exhale, and gradually lengthening your breaths as you feel more relaxed.

8. **Progressive Relaxation**:
- Shut your eyes while you sit or lie down in a comfortable position.
- Starting with your toes, focus on tensing and then relaxing each muscle group in your body, moving gradually from your feet to your head.
- Hold each tension for a few seconds, then release and allow the muscles to relax completely before moving on to the next muscle group.

Practice these relaxation techniques regularly to cultivate a greater sense of calm, reduce stress, and promote overall well-being. Experiment with different techniques to find what works best for you, and remember that consistency is key to experiencing the full benefits of relaxation practice.

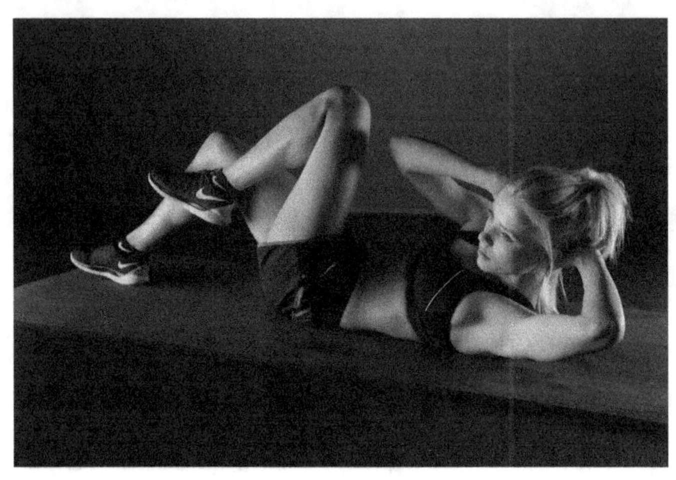

CHAPTER SIX

CREATING A BALANCED MEAL PLAN

Creating a balanced meal plan is essential for individuals looking to manage binge eating disorder (BED) and develop a healthier relationship with food. A balanced meal plan provides a variety of nutrients, helps regulate appetite and energy levels, and supports overall well-being. The following principles can be used to draft a balanced meal plan:

1. **Include a Variety of Nutrient-Rich Foods:**
   - Incorporate a diverse range of foods from all food groups, including fruits, vegetables, whole grains, lean proteins, and healthy fats.
   - Aim for a colorful plate with a variety of fruits and vegetables to maximize nutrient intake and flavor.

2. **Focus on Whole Foods:**
   - Choose whole, minimally processed foods whenever possible, such as whole grains, fresh fruits and vegetables, lean meats, poultry, fish, legumes, nuts, and seeds.
   - Limit the consumption of highly processed and refined foods, such as sugary snacks, baked goods, processed meats, and convenience foods.

3. **Balance Macronutrients**:
   - Aim to include a balance of carbohydrates, proteins, and fats in each meal to promote satiety and provide sustained energy.
   - Carbohydrates: Choose complex carbohydrates such as whole grains, legumes, fruits, and vegetables, which provide fiber and slow-digesting energy.
   - Proteins: Include lean sources of protein such as poultry, fish, tofu, legumes, eggs, and dairy products to support muscle repair and growth.
   - Fats: Incorporate healthy fats from sources such as avocados, nuts, seeds, olive oil, and fatty fish, which provide essential fatty acids and help regulate hormones and inflammation.

4. **Practice Portion Control**:
   - Pay attention to portion sizes and avoid oversized portions, which can lead to overeating.
   - Use measuring cups, spoons, or visual cues to gauge portion sizes and prevent mindless eating.
   - Aim to fill half of your plate with fruits and vegetables, one-quarter with lean protein, and one-quarter with whole grains or starchy vegetables.

5. **Plan Balanced Meals and Snacks**:
   - Plan balanced meals and snacks throughout the day to maintain stable blood sugar levels and prevent excessive hunger or cravings.

- Include a combination of carbohydrates, proteins, and fats in each meal and snack to promote satiety and satisfaction.

- To avoid severe hunger and lessen the chance of binge eating episodes, eat regular meals and snacks at regular intervals throughout the day.

6. **Listen to Your Body**:

- Tune into your body's hunger and fullness cues and eat mindfully, paying attention to physical hunger and satiety signals.

- Eat slowly, chew your food thoroughly, and savor the flavors and textures of each meal to enhance satisfaction and prevent overeating.

- Stop eating when you feel comfortably full and avoid eating past the point of fullness.

7. **Stay Hydrated**:

- Throughout the day, sip on lots of water to stay hydrated and promote general health and wellbeing.

- Limit the consumption of sugary beverages and caffeinated drinks, which can contribute to dehydration and disrupt appetite regulation.

8. **Seek Professional Guidance**:

- Consider consulting with a registered dietitian or nutritionist who specializes in eating disorders or disordered eating patterns for personalized guidance and support in creating a balanced meal plan.

- Work with a healthcare professional to address any underlying medical or nutritional concerns and develop a plan that meets your individual needs and goals.

By following these guidelines and principles, individuals can create a balanced meal plan that supports their nutritional needs, promotes satisfaction and satiety, and contributes to overall health and well-being. Remember that balance, variety, and moderation are key components of a healthy and sustainable approach to eating.

UNDERSTANDING NUTRITIONAL NEEDS

Understanding nutritional needs is crucial for individuals looking to manage binge eating disorder (BED) and promote overall health and well-being. Meeting nutritional needs involves consuming a balanced diet that provides essential nutrients to support bodily functions, energy levels, and overall health. Here are some key aspects to consider when understanding nutritional needs:

1. **Macronutrients**:
   - Carbohydrates: Carbohydrates are the body's primary source of energy and should make up a significant portion of your daily calorie intake. Choose complex carbohydrates such as whole

grains, fruits, vegetables, and legumes, which provide fiber, vitamins, and minerals.

   - Proteins: Proteins are essential for building and repairing tissues, supporting immune function, and maintaining muscle mass. Include lean sources of protein such as poultry, fish, tofu, legumes, eggs, and dairy products in your diet.

   - Fats: Fats are important for hormone production, brain function, and nutrient absorption. Choose healthy fats from sources such as avocados, nuts, seeds, olive oil, and fatty fish, and limit saturated and trans fats found in fried foods, processed snacks, and high-fat meats.

2. **Micronutrients**:

   - Vitamins: Vitamins play essential roles in various bodily functions, including metabolism, immune function, and bone health. Consume a variety of fruits, vegetables, whole grains, and lean proteins to obtain a wide range of vitamins, including vitamin A, vitamin C, vitamin D, vitamin E, and vitamin K.

   - Minerals: Minerals are important for maintaining fluid balance, nerve function, and muscle contractions. Incorporate foods rich in minerals such as calcium, magnesium, potassium, iron, and zinc into your diet, including dairy products, leafy greens, nuts, seeds, and fortified cereals.

   - Trace Elements: Trace elements, such as selenium, copper, iodine, and manganese, are required in smaller amounts but are still essential for overall health and well-being. Include foods such as seafood, nuts, seeds, whole grains, and legumes to ensure adequate intake of trace elements.

3. **Hydration**:
   - Water is essential for maintaining proper hydration, regulating body temperature, and supporting various bodily functions. Drink plenty of water throughout the day, and consume hydrating foods such as fruits, vegetables, and soups to meet your fluid needs.
   - Limit the consumption of sugary beverages, caffeinated drinks, and alcohol, which can contribute to dehydration and disrupt fluid balance.

4. **Energy Needs**:
   - Your energy needs depend on factors such as age, gender, body size, activity level, and metabolic rate. Calculate your daily calorie needs based on these factors and aim to consume a balanced diet that provides adequate energy to support your daily activities and bodily functions.
   - Be mindful of portion sizes and avoid overeating or undereating, which can lead to fluctuations in energy levels and contribute to binge eating episodes.

5. **Individual Variability**:
   - Nutritional needs vary from person to person based on factors such as age, gender, genetics, health status, and lifestyle factors. Consider your unique needs and preferences when planning your

diet and consult with a registered dietitian or nutritionist for personalized guidance and support.

   - Be mindful of any dietary restrictions, food allergies, or medical conditions that may impact your nutritional needs and make adjustments to your diet as needed to ensure optimal health and well-being.

Understanding your nutritional needs and making informed diet decisions is vital for managing binge eating disorder and promoting general health and well-being. Focus on consuming a balanced diet that includes a variety of nutrient-rich foods, stays hydrated, and supports your individual needs and goals for optimal health and well-being.

PLANNING BALANCED MEALS AND SNACKS

Planning balanced meals and snacks is essential for managing binge eating disorder (BED) and promoting overall health and well-being. Balanced meals and snacks provide a combination of macronutrients (carbohydrates, proteins, and fats), essential vitamins and minerals, and fiber to support energy levels, satiety, and overall nutrition. Here are some tips for planning balanced meals and snacks:

1. **Include a Variety of Food Groups**:

- Aim to include foods from all food groups in your meals and snacks to ensure a diverse and nutrient-rich diet.
- Choose a variety of fruits, vegetables, whole grains, lean proteins, and healthy fats to provide essential nutrients and promote overall health.

2. **Balance Macronutrients**:
- Each meal and snack should contain a balance of carbohydrates, proteins, and fats to promote satiety, stabilize blood sugar levels, and support overall nutrition.
- Carbohydrates: Choose complex carbohydrates such as whole grains, fruits, vegetables, and legumes, which provide fiber, vitamins, and minerals.
- Proteins: Include lean sources of protein such as poultry, fish, tofu, legumes, eggs, and dairy products to support muscle repair and growth.
- Fats: Incorporate healthy fats from sources such as avocados, nuts, seeds, olive oil, and fatty fish to support heart health, brain function, and hormone production.

3. **Portion Control**:
- Be mindful of portion sizes and steer clear of excessive portions, which can cause discomfort and overindulgence.
- Use measuring cups, spoons, or visual cues to gauge portion sizes and prevent mindless eating.
- Aim to fill half of your plate with fruits and vegetables, one-quarter with lean protein, and

one-quarter with whole grains or starchy vegetables.

4. **Plan Ahead**:
   - Take time to plan your meals and snacks in advance to ensure you have nutritious options available throughout the day.
   - Consider preparing meals and snacks ahead of time, such as batch cooking and portioning out servings for quick and convenient options during busy times.

5. **Include Fiber-Rich Foods**:
   - Incorporate fiber-rich foods such as fruits, vegetables, whole grains, legumes, nuts, and seeds into your meals and snacks to promote digestive health, regulate appetite, and support weight management.
   - Aim to include a variety of fiber sources throughout the day to meet your daily fiber needs and promote satiety.

6. **Stay Hydrated**:
   - Throughout the day, sip on lots of water to stay hydrated and promote general health and wellbeing.
   - Include hydrating foods such as fruits, vegetables, and soups in your meals and snacks to help meet your fluid needs.

7. **Listen to Your Body**:

- Tune into your body's hunger and fullness cues and eat mindfully, paying attention to physical hunger and satiety signals.
- Eat slowly, chew your food thoroughly, and savor the flavors and textures of each meal to enhance satisfaction and prevent overeating.
- Stop eating when you feel comfortably full and avoid eating past the point of fullness.

By planning balanced meals and snacks that include a variety of nutrient-rich foods, you can support your nutritional needs, promote satiety and satisfaction, and contribute to overall health and well-being. Experiment with different meal and snack combinations, listen to your body's cues, and make adjustments as needed to find a balanced eating pattern that works for you.

INCORPORATING VARIETY AND FLEXIBILITY

Incorporating variety and flexibility into your meal planning and eating habits is essential for managing binge eating disorder (BED) and promoting a healthy relationship with food. Variety and flexibility allow for enjoyment, satisfaction, and adaptability in your diet while still meeting your nutritional needs. Here's how to incorporate variety and flexibility into your approach:

1. **Explore Different Foods**:

- Experiment with new foods, flavors, and recipes to keep your meals interesting and enjoyable.
- Try incorporating a variety of fruits, vegetables, whole grains, lean proteins, and healthy fats into your meals to provide a diverse range of nutrients and flavors.

2. **Rotate Meals and Snacks**:
- Rotate your meals and snacks regularly to avoid monotony and ensure you're getting a variety of nutrients throughout the week.
- Plan different meals and snacks each day or week to keep things fresh and exciting, and allow yourself the flexibility to change things up based on your preferences and cravings.

3. **Include Cultural and Ethnic Foods**:
- Embrace the diversity of cultural and ethnic cuisines by incorporating dishes from different cultures into your meal rotation.
- Explore recipes and cooking techniques from around the world to add new flavors, textures, and culinary experiences to your diet.

4. **Modify Recipes and Meals**:
- Modify recipes and meals to suit your preferences, dietary needs, and ingredient availability.
- Feel free to swap ingredients, adjust portion sizes, or customize recipes to make them more nutritious or better suited to your taste preferences.

5. **Practice Intuitive Eating**:
   - Practice intuitive eating by listening to your body's hunger and fullness cues, and eating based on your individual needs and preferences.
   - Allow yourself to enjoy a wide variety of foods in moderation without labeling them as "good" or "bad," and focus on honoring your hunger, fullness, and satisfaction.

6. **Allow for Flexibility**:
   - Be flexible with your meal planning and eating habits, and allow yourself the freedom to respond to changes in your schedule, cravings, or social situations.
   - Don't be too rigid or restrictive with your food choices, and allow for occasional indulgences or treats without guilt or shame.

7. **Embrace Seasonal and Local Foods**:
   - Embrace seasonal and local foods by incorporating fresh produce that's in season into your meals and snacks.
   - Visit farmers' markets or join a community-supported agriculture (CSA) program to discover seasonal and locally grown foods and support sustainable agriculture practices.

8. **Practice Mindful Eating**:
   - Practice mindful eating by savoring each bite, paying attention to the flavors, textures, and sensations of the food, and eating without distractions.

- Slow down and tune into your body's hunger and fullness cues, and make conscious choices about what, when, and how much to eat based on your body's needs.

By incorporating variety and flexibility into your meal planning and eating habits, you can enjoy a diverse and satisfying diet while still meeting your nutritional needs and supporting your overall health and well-being. Experiment with different foods, flavors, and recipes, and find a balanced and flexible approach to eating that works for you.

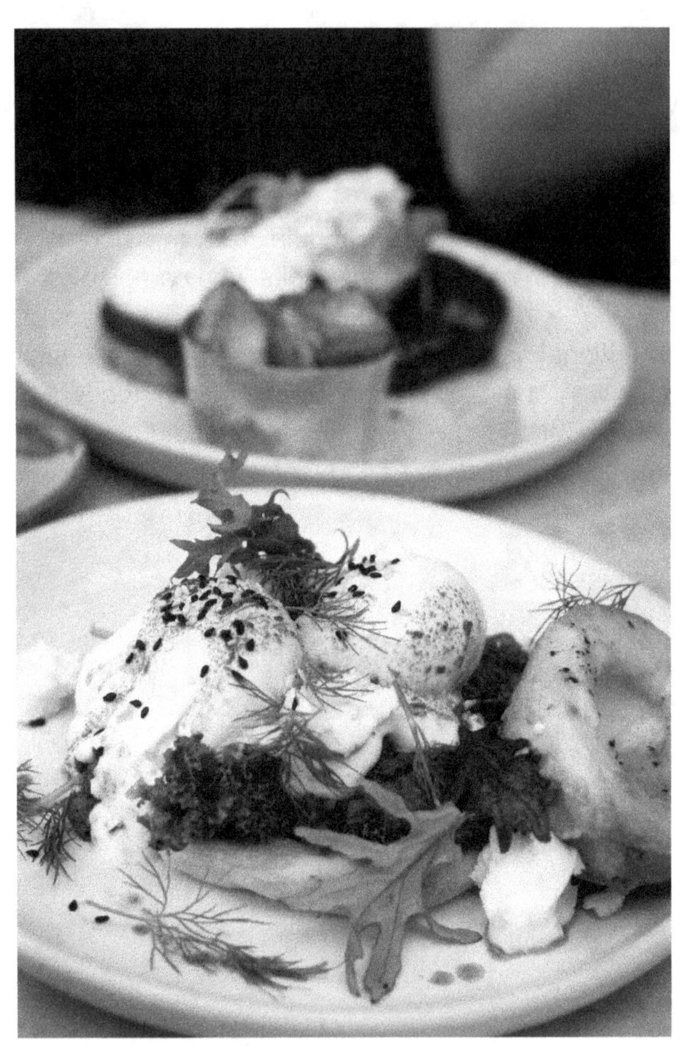

CHAPTER SEVEN

BREAKING THE BINGE CYCLE

Breaking the binge cycle is a crucial step in managing binge eating disorder (BED) and establishing a healthier relationship with food. While it can be difficult to stop the cycle, there are methods and strategies that can assist people in overcoming periods of binge eating and adopting better eating practices. Here are some tips for breaking the binge cycle:

1. **Identify Triggers**: Recognize the emotional, environmental, and physiological triggers that contribute to binge eating episodes. Common triggers may include stress, boredom, negative emotions, social situations, or restrictive eating patterns.

2. **Develop Coping Strategies**: Learn healthy coping strategies to manage triggers and reduce the urge to binge eat. Practice stress management techniques, such as deep breathing, mindfulness, meditation, or engaging in enjoyable activities, to cope with difficult emotions and situations without turning to food.

3. **Practice Mindful Eating**: Cultivate awareness and mindfulness around eating by paying attention to hunger and fullness cues, eating

slowly, and savoring the flavors and textures of food. Practice mindful eating to tune into your body's signals and make conscious choices about when, what, and how much to eat.

4. **Address Emotional Needs**: Explore underlying emotional needs and address them through self-care, therapy, or support from friends and family. Seek professional help if needed to work through emotional issues and develop healthier coping mechanisms for managing emotions.

5. **Avoid Restrictive Dieting**: Avoid restrictive dieting or extreme food rules, as they can contribute to feelings of deprivation, binge eating, and an unhealthy relationship with food. Focus on nourishing your body with balanced meals and snacks that include a variety of nutrient-rich foods.

6. **Practice Self-Compassion**: Be kind and compassionate towards yourself, especially during challenging times or after a binge eating episode. Practice self-compassion by acknowledging your struggles, forgiving yourself for setbacks, and focusing on progress rather than perfection.

7. **Seek Support**: Reach out for support from friends, family members, or support groups who can offer empathy, understanding, and encouragement. Consider joining a support group or seeking therapy from a mental health

professional who specializes in treating binge eating disorder.

8. **Challenge Negative Thoughts:** Challenge negative thoughts and beliefs about yourself, your body, and food that contribute to the binge cycle. Replace negative self-talk with more balanced and compassionate perspectives, and work on developing a positive body image and self-esteem.

9. **Create a Supportive Environment:** Surround yourself with a supportive environment that promotes healthy eating habits and positive self-care. Stock your kitchen with nutritious foods, remove triggers or temptations for binge eating, and cultivate a supportive network of friends and loved ones.

10. **Practice Persistence and Patience:** Breaking the binge cycle takes time, patience, and persistence. Be gentle with yourself and acknowledge your minor accomplishments along the way. Remember that recovery is a journey, and every step forward is a step towards healing and well-being.

By implementing these strategies and techniques, individuals can break the binge cycle, regain control over their eating habits, and work towards establishing a healthier and more balanced relationship with food. It's important to seek support, practice self-care, and be patient with yourself throughout the recovery process.

STRATEGIES FOR INTERRUPTING BINGE EPISODES

Interrupting binge episodes is a crucial skill for individuals managing binge eating disorder (BED) to regain control over their eating habits and prevent further escalation. The following techniques can be used to stop binge episodes:

1. **Pause and Breathe**: When you feel the urge to binge, take a moment to pause and take a few deep breaths. Focus on slowing down your breathing and calming your mind before taking any further action.

2. **Distract Yourself**: Engage in a distracting activity to shift your focus away from food and the urge to binge. Try going for a walk, calling a friend, doing a puzzle, listening to music, or engaging in a hobby or activity that you enjoy.

3. **Remove Temptations**: Remove or distance yourself from binge-triggering foods to reduce the temptation to overeat. Clear your environment of trigger foods, such as sweets, snacks, or processed foods, and keep them out of sight or out of reach.

4. **Practice Mindfulness**: Practice mindfulness techniques to increase awareness of your thoughts, emotions, and bodily sensations without judgment. Observe the urge to binge with curiosity and detachment, allowing it to pass without acting on it.

5. **Delay the Binge**: Delay acting on the urge to binge by setting a timer for 10-15 minutes and waiting before making a decision. Use this time to reassess your feelings, engage in a distracting activity, or practice mindfulness to ride out the urge.

6. **Challenge Negative Thoughts**: Challenge negative thoughts and beliefs that contribute to the urge to binge. Question the validity of thoughts such as "I can't control myself" or "I'll feel better if I eat," and replace them with more balanced and rational perspectives.

7. **Reach Out for Support**: When you find yourself fighting with the impulse to binge, ask a trusted friend, family member, or support group for assistance. Share your feelings and experiences with someone who can offer empathy, understanding, and encouragement.

8. **Use Coping Strategies**: Use healthy coping strategies to manage emotions and stressors that trigger binge eating. To ease tension and anxiety, try relaxation techniques like progressive muscle relaxation, deep breathing, or meditation.

9. **Create a Binge Box:** Create a "binge box" filled with non-food items that provide comfort and distraction during moments of distress. Fill the box with items such as stress balls, sensory toys, coloring books, or soothing teas to use as alternative coping tools.

10. **Seek Professional Help:** If binge episodes persist despite your efforts to interrupt them, seek professional help from a therapist, counselor, or healthcare provider who specializes in treating binge eating disorder. Professional support can provide additional coping strategies, guidance, and accountability in managing binge episodes.

Remember that interrupting binge episodes takes practice and persistence, and it's okay to seek support when needed. Be patient and compassionate with yourself as you work towards developing healthier coping mechanisms and overcoming binge eating behaviors.

COPING WITH SLIP-UPS AND STEP BACK

One of the most crucial aspects of treating binge eating disorder (BED) and continuing the healing process is learning to cope with mistakes and failures. Slip-ups and steps back are a natural part of the journey, and it's essential to approach them with compassion, understanding, and a willingness to learn and grow. Here are some strategies for coping with slip-ups and setbacks:

1. **Practice Self-Compassion**: Be gentle and kind with yourself when experiencing a slip-up or setback. Recognize that setbacks are a normal part of the recovery process and that you're not alone in experiencing them. Give yourself the same compassion and understanding that you would extend to a buddy in a comparable circumstance.

2. **Avoid Self-Blame and Guilt**: Refrain from blaming yourself or feeling guilty for slipping up. Instead of dwelling on past mistakes, focus on what you can learn from the experience and how you can move forward in a positive direction. Remind yourself that slip-ups do not define your worth or your ability to recover.

3. **Learn from the Experience**: Reflect on the factors that contributed to the slip-up or setback and identify any triggers, emotions, or situations that may have played a role. Use the experience as an opportunity to gain insight into your patterns of behavior and develop strategies for preventing similar situations in the future.

4. **Reframe Negative Thoughts**: Challenge negative thoughts and beliefs that arise after a slip-up or setback. Replace self-critical or defeatist thoughts with more balanced and constructive perspectives. For example, instead of thinking, "I'm

a failure," remind yourself that setbacks are temporary and that you have the strength and resilience to overcome challenges.

5. **Focus on Progress, Not Perfection**: Shift your focus from perfectionism to progress by acknowledging the positive steps you've taken towards recovery. Celebrate small victories and milestones along the way, no matter how minor they may seem. Remember that recovery is a journey, and setbacks are opportunities for growth and learning.

6. **Recommit to Your Goals**: Reaffirm your commitment to recovery and your long-term goals for health and well-being. Use the setback as motivation to recommit to positive habits and behaviors that support your recovery journey. Set realistic and achievable goals for yourself, and take proactive steps towards reaching them.

7. **Seek Support**: Reach out for support from friends, family members, or support groups who can offer empathy, encouragement, and understanding during challenging times. Share your feelings and experiences with someone you trust, and lean on your support network for guidance and validation.

8. **Practice Coping Skills**: Use coping skills and strategies to manage difficult emotions and prevent future slip-ups. Practice stress

management techniques, engage in self-care activities, and develop healthy coping mechanisms for dealing with triggers and cravings.

9. **Stay Flexible and Adaptive**: Stay flexible and adaptable in your approach to recovery, and be willing to adjust your strategies as needed based on your experiences and feedback. Accept the process of making mistakes and be willing to attempt novel methods and strategies for controlling your binge eating habits.

10. **Seek Professional Help if Needed**: If slip-ups and setbacks become overwhelming or persistent, consider seeking professional help from a therapist, counselor, or healthcare provider who specializes in treating binge eating disorder. Professional support can provide additional guidance, coping strategies, and resources to support your recovery journey.

Remember that slip-ups and setbacks are a normal part of the recovery process, and they do not diminish your progress or your potential for success. Approach them with patience, self-compassion, and a willingness to learn, and use them as opportunities for growth and self-discovery on your journey towards recovery from binge eating disorder.

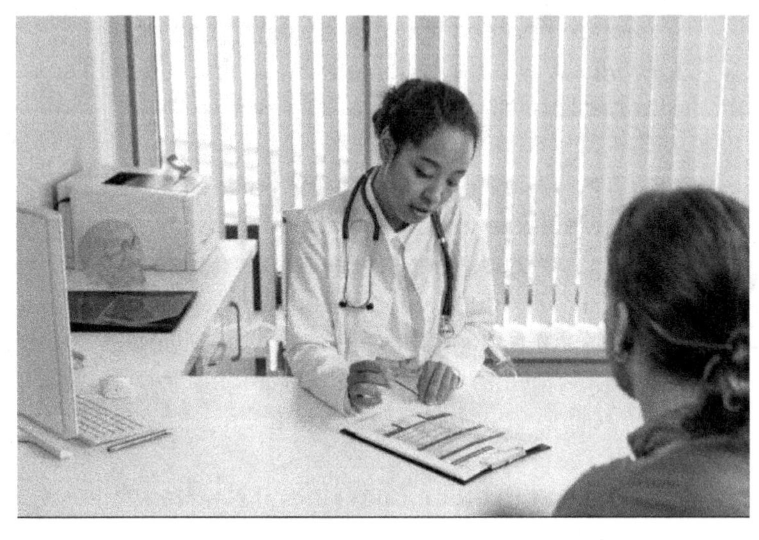

CHAPTER EIGHT

ADDRESSING UNDERLYING ISSUES

One of the most important aspects of treating binge eating disorder (BED) and encouraging long-term recovery is addressing underlying concerns. Underlying issues can contribute to the development and maintenance of BED, and addressing them is essential for understanding and treating the root causes of disordered eating behaviors. Here are some strategies for addressing underlying issues:

1. **Identify Triggers and Patterns**: Take time to identify the emotional, environmental, and psychological triggers that contribute to binge eating episodes. Keep a journal to track your thoughts, feelings, and behaviors around food, and look for patterns or common triggers that precede binge eating episodes.

2. **Explore Past Experiences**: Reflect on past experiences, traumas, or events that may have contributed to the development of disordered eating behaviors. Consider how early life experiences, relationships, family dynamics, or cultural influences may have shaped your relationship with food and your body.

3. **Seek Professional Help**: Consider seeking professional help from a therapist, counselor, or healthcare provider who specializes in treating eating disorders. A trained professional can help you explore underlying issues, process difficult emotions, and develop coping strategies for managing triggers and cravings.

4. **Therapy and Counseling**: Participate in individual therapy, counseling, or psychotherapy to address underlying issues and develop healthier coping mechanisms. Cognitive-behavioral therapy (CBT), dialectical behavior therapy (DBT), interpersonal therapy (IPT), and other evidence-based approaches can be effective in treating binge eating disorder.

5. **Address Co-occurring Disorders**: Address any co-occurring mental health disorders or conditions that may be contributing to binge eating behaviors, such as depression, anxiety, trauma, or substance abuse. Work with a healthcare provider to develop a comprehensive treatment plan that addresses all aspects of your mental and emotional well-being.

6. **Explore Family Dynamics**: Examine family dynamics and relationships that may influence your eating behaviors and body image. Consider how family history, communication patterns, and

interpersonal dynamics may impact your relationship with food and your body image.

7. **Practice Self-Reflection**: Engage in self-reflection and introspection to better understand your thoughts, feelings, and behaviors surrounding food and eating. Take time to explore your values, beliefs, and motivations related to food, body image, and self-esteem.

8. **Develop Coping Skills**: Learn healthy coping skills and strategies for managing stress, emotions, and triggers without turning to food. Practice relaxation techniques, mindfulness, stress management, and emotion regulation skills to build resilience and enhance coping abilities.

9. **Build Support Networks**: Surround yourself with supportive friends, family members, or support groups who can offer empathy, understanding, and encouragement on your journey to recovery. Share your experiences, struggles, and successes with others who can relate and provide validation and support.

10. **Take Small Steps**: Take small, manageable steps towards addressing underlying issues and improving your relationship with food and your body. Set realistic goals for yourself, and celebrate progress and achievements along the way, no matter how small they may seem.

Addressing underlying issues is a complex and ongoing process that requires patience, self-awareness, and commitment. Be gentle with yourself as you explore and work through underlying issues, and remember that recovery from binge eating disorder is possible with support, dedication, and perseverance.

EXPLORING POTENTIAL UNDERLYING CAUSES OF BINGE EATING

Exploring potential underlying causes of binge eating can provide insight into the factors contributing to disordered eating behaviors and inform effective treatment strategies. While the causes of binge eating disorder (BED) can vary from person to person, there are several common underlying factors that may contribute to the development and maintenance of binge eating behaviors. Here are some potential underlying causes to explore:

1. **Emotional Factors**:
   - **Stress**: High levels of stress, whether from work, relationships, financial pressures, or other sources, can trigger binge eating as a way to cope with or numb difficult emotions.
   - **Trauma**: Past experiences of trauma, abuse, neglect, or significant life events can contribute to disordered eating behaviors as a means of coping

with unresolved emotional pain or trauma-related symptoms.

   - **Negative Emotions**: Feelings of sadness, loneliness, anxiety, depression, or low self-esteem can lead to binge eating as a way to self-soothe, distract from emotional discomfort, or seek temporary relief.

2. **Psychological Factors**:

   - **Perfectionism**: Unrealistic standards of perfection or a fear of failure can contribute to binge eating behaviors as individuals strive to control their emotions or alleviate feelings of inadequacy.

   - **Body Image Disturbance**: Negative body image, dissatisfaction with one's appearance, or internalized societal pressures to achieve an ideal body shape or size can fuel binge eating behaviors as individuals attempt to cope with body-related distress.

   - **Dysfunctional Coping Mechanisms**: Difficulty regulating emotions, managing stress, or coping with difficult situations can lead to maladaptive coping mechanisms, such as binge eating, as a way to manage overwhelming emotions or situations.

3. **Environmental Factors**:

   - **Food Environment**: Access to highly palatable, calorie-dense foods, frequent exposure to food-related cues or triggers, and social norms that encourage overeating can contribute to binge eating behaviors.

- **Family Dynamics**: Family history of disordered eating, dysfunctional family relationships, or a lack of emotional support or communication within the family environment can impact an individual's relationship with food and eating behaviors.
- **Cultural Influences**: Cultural attitudes towards food, body image, weight, and eating behaviors can shape an individual's beliefs, behaviors, and attitudes surrounding food and eating.

4. **Biological Factors**:
- **Genetics**: Genetic predisposition or family history of eating disorders, obesity, or mental health conditions may increase susceptibility to developing binge eating disorder.
- **Neurobiology**: Alterations in brain chemistry, neurotransmitter imbalances, or dysfunction in reward pathways involved in food intake, pleasure, and self-regulation may contribute to binge eating behaviors.

5. **Interpersonal Factors**:
- **Social Pressures**: Social pressures to conform to diet culture, body ideals, or societal expectations regarding food and weight can influence an individual's eating behaviors and body image.
- **Relationship Issues**: Dysfunctional or strained relationships, conflict, lack of social support, or a history of interpersonal trauma can

impact an individual's emotional well-being and contribute to binge eating behaviors as a coping mechanism.

Exploring these potential underlying causes of binge eating can help individuals gain insight into the factors contributing to their disordered eating behaviors and inform personalized treatment approaches. It's important to approach exploration with curiosity, compassion, and openness to understanding the complex interplay of factors that contribute to binge eating disorder. Seeking support from a therapist, counselor, or healthcare provider who specializes in eating disorders can provide guidance, validation, and resources for addressing underlying causes and promoting recovery.

SEEKING PROFESSIONAL HELP FOR CO-OCCURRING DISORDERS

For those who are treating binge eating disorder (BED) in addition to other mental health concerns, getting professional assistance for co-occurring disorders is imperative. Co-occurring disorders, such as depression, anxiety, trauma-related disorders, substance use disorders, or other eating disorders, can complicate the treatment process and impact overall well-being. Here are some steps for seeking professional help for co-occurring disorders:

1. **Assessment and Diagnosis**: Seek an assessment and diagnosis from a qualified healthcare provider, such as a psychiatrist, psychologist, therapist, or primary care physician, to determine the presence of co-occurring disorders. Describe your symptoms, experiences, and concerns openly and honestly to facilitate an accurate diagnosis.

2. **Treatment Planning**: Collaborate with your healthcare provider to develop a comprehensive treatment plan that addresses all co-occurring disorders simultaneously. Consider the unique needs, challenges, and goals associated with each disorder, and tailor treatment interventions accordingly.

3. **Integrated Treatment Approach**: Choose an integrated treatment approach that combines evidence-based interventions for binge eating disorder and co-occurring disorders. Integrated treatment models, such as dialectical behavior therapy (DBT), cognitive-behavioral therapy (CBT), or trauma-informed care, address the complex interplay of factors contributing to both disorders.

4. **Medication Management**: Discuss medication options with your healthcare provider for managing symptoms of co-occurring disorders, such as depression, anxiety, or mood disturbances. Medication may be prescribed in conjunction with

therapy or counseling to support symptom management and overall recovery.

5. **Therapy and Counseling**: Participate in individual therapy, counseling, or psychotherapy to address underlying issues, develop coping skills, and learn strategies for managing symptoms of co-occurring disorders. Choose a therapist or counselor who specializes in treating both binge eating disorder and co-occurring mental health conditions.

6. **Group Therapy or Support Groups**: Consider participating in group therapy or support groups specifically tailored to individuals with co-occurring disorders. Group therapy provides opportunities for peer support, validation, and shared experiences, and can complement individual therapy in promoting recovery.

7. **Specialized Treatment Programs**: Explore specialized treatment programs or clinics that offer comprehensive care for individuals with co-occurring disorders. Look for programs that provide multidisciplinary treatment teams, evidence-based interventions, and a supportive therapeutic environment conducive to healing and recovery.

8. **Continued Monitoring and Follow-Up**: Maintain regular communication with your healthcare providers and participate in ongoing monitoring and follow-up to track progress, address challenges, and adjust treatment as needed. Be proactive in advocating for your needs and seeking additional support or resources when necessary.

9. **Self-Care and Support**: Prioritize self-care practices, such as adequate sleep, nutrition, physical activity, and stress management, to support overall well-being and recovery from co-occurring disorders. Lean on your support network of friends, family members, or support groups for encouragement, validation, and empathy during difficult times.

10. **Be Patient and Persistent**: Recovery from co-occurring disorders takes time, patience, and persistence. Be gentle with yourself as you navigate the treatment process, and celebrate small victories and milestones along the way. Remember that progress is nonlinear, and setbacks are a natural part of the journey towards healing and recovery.

Seeking professional help for co-occurring disorders is an important step towards addressing underlying issues, promoting holistic healing, and fostering long-term recovery from binge eating disorder and other mental health conditions. Be proactive in advocating for your well-being and accessing the resources and support you need to thrive.

WORKING THROUGH PAST TRAUMAS OR TRIGGERS

Working through past traumas or triggers is an essential aspect of managing binge eating disorder (BED) and promoting healing and recovery. Trauma and triggers can significantly impact an individual's relationship with food, body image, and eating behaviors, and addressing these underlying issues is crucial for developing healthier coping mechanisms and lowering binge eating episodes' frequency and intensity. Here are some strategies for working through past traumas or triggers:

1. **Seek Professional Help**: Consider seeking professional help from a therapist, counselor, or mental health professional who specializes in trauma-informed care and eating disorders. A trained therapist can provide a safe and supportive environment for exploring past traumas, processing difficult emotions, and developing coping strategies for managing triggers.

2. **Trauma-Informed Therapy**: Participate in trauma-informed therapy or modalities specifically designed to address trauma-related issues, such as eye movement desensitization and reprocessing (EMDR), cognitive processing therapy (CPT), or narrative therapy. These approaches can help individuals process traumatic memories, reframe negative beliefs, and promote healing from past traumas.

3. **Mindfulness and Grounding Techniques**:
Practice mindfulness and grounding techniques to
help manage distressing emotions and sensations
associated with past traumas or triggers. Engage in
deep breathing exercises, progressive muscle
relaxation, guided imagery, or sensory grounding
techniques to promote relaxation and
present-moment awareness.

4. **Emotional Regulation Skills**: Learn
emotional regulation skills to cope with intense
emotions triggered by past traumas. Practice
identifying and labeling emotions, expressing
feelings in healthy ways, and developing strategies
for self-soothing and calming during times of
distress.

5. **Identify Triggers**: Identify specific triggers or
cues that elicit binge eating episodes related to
past traumas. Track the events, feelings, ideas, and
actions that lead to binge eating episodes in your
diary. Then, look for trends or recurring triggers that
support disordered eating behaviors.

6. **Cognitive Restructuring**: Challenge and
reframe negative beliefs or thought patterns
associated with past traumas or triggers. Replace
distorted or maladaptive thoughts with more
balanced and adaptive perspectives, and develop a
compassionate and nurturing inner dialogue.

7. **Create a Safety Plan**: Develop a safety plan or coping strategy for managing triggers and cravings related to past traumas. Establish a plan for controlling cravings to binge eat, as well as healthy coping strategies, social supports, and self-care routines that you can rely on in trying times.

8. **Build Resilience**: Cultivate resilience and inner strength by focusing on your strengths, values, and sources of support. Practice self-compassion, self-care, and self-acceptance as you navigate the process of healing from past traumas and building a healthier relationship with food and your body.

9. **Set Boundaries**: Establish healthy boundaries in your relationships and environments to protect yourself from retraumatization or exposure to triggering situations. Advocate for your needs, communicate assertively, and prioritize your emotional well-being in your interactions with others.

10. **Practice Patience and Self-Care**: Be patient with yourself as you work through past traumas or triggers and prioritize self-care practices that support your healing journey. Take breaks when needed, engage in activities that bring you joy and fulfillment, and celebrate your progress and accomplishments along the way.

Working through past traumas or triggers is a gradual and ongoing process that requires patience, courage, and self-compassion. By seeking professional help, developing coping skills, and building resilience, individuals can gradually heal from past traumas, reduce the impact of triggers on their eating behaviors, and cultivate a healthier relationship with food and their bodies.

CHAPTER NINE

LONG-TERM MAINTENANCE

Long-term maintenance is a crucial aspect of managing binge eating disorder (BED) and promoting sustained recovery and well-being. While overcoming binge eating behaviors is an important milestone, maintaining progress and preventing relapse requires ongoing effort, commitment, and self-care. Here are some strategies for long-term maintenance:

1. **Consistent Self-Care**: Prioritize self-care practices that support your physical, emotional, and mental well-being on a regular basis. This includes adequate sleep, nutritious eating, regular physical activity, stress management, and engaging in activities that bring you joy and fulfillment.

2. **Mindful Eating**: Continue practicing mindful eating techniques to stay attuned to your body's hunger and fullness cues, as well as your emotional and psychological relationship with food. Eat slowly, savor your meals, and pay attention to how different foods make you feel physically and emotionally.

3. **Regular Monitoring**: Stay vigilant about monitoring your thoughts, feelings, and behaviors surrounding food and eating. Keep a journal to

track your eating patterns, emotional triggers, and stress levels, and be proactive in addressing any warning signs of relapse or distress.

4. **Healthy Coping Mechanisms**: Develop and maintain healthy coping mechanisms for managing stress, emotions, and triggers without turning to food. Practice relaxation techniques, seek support from friends or family, engage in hobbies or activities you enjoy, and consider professional help if needed.

5. **Social Support**: Cultivate a strong support network of friends, family members, or support groups who understand and validate your experiences with BED. Stay connected with others who share similar struggles and provide encouragement, empathy, and accountability in your recovery journey.

6. **Regular Therapy or Counseling**: Continue participating in therapy, counseling, or support groups to address underlying issues, learn coping skills, and maintain accountability in your recovery. Regular check-ins with a mental health professional can help prevent relapse and provide ongoing guidance and support.

7. **Flexible Meal Planning**: Maintain a balanced and flexible approach to meal planning and eating, focusing on nourishing your body with a variety of nutrient-rich foods while also allowing for

occasional indulgences or treats. Avoid rigid dieting or restrictive eating patterns that may trigger binge eating behaviors.

8. **Stress Management**: Prioritize stress management techniques and strategies to reduce the impact of stress on your eating behaviors and overall well-being. Practice mindfulness, deep breathing, yoga, meditation, or other stress-reduction techniques to promote relaxation and resilience.

9. **Continued Education and Learning**: Stay informed about BED, eating disorders, mental health, and self-care by seeking out reliable sources of information, attending workshops or seminars, or reading books and articles on related topics. Continuously educate yourself and remain open to learning new strategies for maintaining recovery.

10. **Celebrate Milestones**: Acknowledge and celebrate your progress and achievements along the way, no matter how small they may seem. Set realistic goals for yourself, and take pride in the steps you've taken towards healing and recovery from BED.

Long-term maintenance of recovery from binge eating disorder requires dedication, perseverance, and a commitment to self-care and self-awareness. By implementing these strategies and remaining

vigilant about your physical and emotional
well-being, you can sustain your progress and
enjoy a fulfilling life free from the grip of binge
eating behaviors. Remember that recovery is a
journey, and each day presents an opportunity for
growth, healing, and renewal.

SETTING REALISTIC GOALS

In order to manage binge eating disorder (BED)
and encourage sustained progress towards
recovery, it is imperative to set realistic goals.
Realistic goals are achievable, meaningful, and
tailored to your individual needs, abilities, and
circumstances. Here are some tips for setting
realistic goals in the context of BED:

1. **Assess Your Current Situation**: Take stock
of your current eating habits, emotional well-being,
physical health, and overall quality of life. Identify
areas where you'd like to see improvement or
change, and consider how these goals align with
your values and priorities.

2. **Break Down Goals into Manageable
Steps**: Divide larger, long-term goals into smaller,
more manageable steps or milestones. Break down
your goals into specific actions or behaviors that
you can work on gradually over time, making
progress more achievable and sustainable.

3. **Set SMART Goals**: Use the SMART criteria to structure your goals:
   - **Specific**: Make sure your goals are well-defined.
   - **Measurable**: Include criteria for measuring progress and success.
   - **Achievable**: Ensure that your goals are realistic and attainable given your resources and limitations.
   - **Relevant**: Make sure your goals are relevant to your values, priorities, and overall well-being.
   - **Time-bound**: Set deadlines or timeframes for achieving your goals to create a sense of urgency and accountability.

4. **Focus on Behavioral Changes**: Shift your focus from outcome-based goals (e.g., losing a certain amount of weight) to behavior-based goals (e.g., practicing mindful eating, engaging in regular physical activity). Emphasize actions and behaviors that you have control over and can actively work on.

5. **Prioritize Self-Care**: Include self-care goals as part of your overall plan for managing BED. Prioritize activities and practices that support your physical, emotional, and mental well-being, such as getting enough sleep, eating nourishing meals, practicing relaxation techniques, and engaging in enjoyable activities.

6. **Be Flexible and Adaptive**: Remain flexible and open to adjusting your goals as needed based on your progress, feedback, and changing circumstances. Be willing to reassess and revise your goals over time to ensure they remain relevant and achievable.

7. **Celebrate Progress**: Acknowledge and celebrate your progress and achievements, no matter how small. Celebrating milestones along the way can boost motivation, reinforce positive behaviors, and provide encouragement to continue moving forward.

8. **Seek Support and Accountability**: Share your goals with supportive friends, family members, or healthcare providers who can offer encouragement, validation, and accountability. Consider joining a support group or seeking guidance from a therapist who specializes in treating BED.

9. **Practice Self-Compassion**: Be kind and compassionate with yourself as you work towards your goals. Accept that setbacks and challenges are a natural part of the process, and treat yourself with the same empathy and understanding that you would offer to a friend in a similar situation.

10. **Stay Committed and Persistent**: Stay committed to your goals and remain persistent in your efforts, even when faced with obstacles or

setbacks. Remember that progress takes time and effort, and stay focused on the long-term benefits of investing in your health and well-being.

By setting realistic goals that are specific, measurable, achievable, relevant, and time-bound, you can create a roadmap for managing BED and promoting lasting recovery. Focus on making gradual, sustainable changes, prioritizing self-care, and seeking support when needed. With dedication, patience, and perseverance, you can work towards achieving your goals and enjoying a healthier relationship with food and your body.

MONITORING PROGRESS AND MAKING ADJUSTMENTS

Monitoring progress and making adjustments are essential components of managing binge eating disorder (BED) and promoting long-term recovery. Regularly assessing your progress allows you to track your achievements, identify areas for improvement, and make necessary changes to your treatment plan. Here are some strategies for effectively monitoring progress and making adjustments in the context of BED:

1. **Set Clear Goals**: Establish clear, specific, and measurable goals for managing BED and improving your overall well-being. Clearly defined

goals provide a framework for monitoring progress and evaluating success.

2. **Track Behaviors and Symptoms**: Keep track of your eating behaviors, binge episodes, emotional triggers, and symptoms of BED on a regular basis. Use a journal, diary, or tracking app to record relevant information and identify patterns over time.

3. **Use Assessment Tools**: Utilize standardized assessment tools or questionnaires designed to evaluate symptoms of BED, such as the Binge Eating Scale (BES) or the Eating Disorder Examination Questionnaire (EDE-Q). These tools can help quantify symptoms, track changes over time, and inform treatment decisions.

4. **Regular Check-Ins**: Schedule regular check-ins with your healthcare provider, therapist, or treatment team to review your progress and discuss any challenges or concerns. These appointments provide an opportunity to receive feedback, adjust treatment goals, and make necessary modifications to your treatment plan.

5. **Evaluate Strategies and Interventions**: Assess the effectiveness of strategies and interventions implemented to manage BED, such as therapy, medication, self-help techniques, or lifestyle changes. Evaluate which approaches are

helping you make progress towards your goals and which may need to be modified or discontinued.

6. **Identify Triggers and Patterns**: Identify triggers, stressors, or situations that contribute to binge eating episodes or interfere with your progress. Recognize patterns in your behavior, emotions, and environment that may impact your ability to manage BED effectively.

7. **Seek Feedback**: Seek feedback from trusted friends, family members, or support group members who can provide perspective on your progress and offer insights into areas for improvement. External feedback can offer valuable insights and validation as you work towards recovery.

8. **Be Flexible and Adaptive**: Remain flexible and open to making adjustments to your treatment plan based on your evolving needs and circumstances. Be willing to experiment with different strategies, approaches, and interventions to find what works best for you.

9. **Celebrate Progress**: Acknowledge and celebrate your achievements, milestones, and successes along the way. Celebrating progress, no matter how small, can boost motivation, reinforce positive behaviors, and provide encouragement to continue moving forward.

10. **Practice Self-Reflection**: Take time for self-reflection to assess your progress, identify barriers or obstacles, and explore opportunities for growth and improvement. Regular self-reflection promotes self-awareness and empowers you to make informed decisions about your treatment and recovery journey.

By consistently monitoring your progress, identifying areas for improvement, and making necessary adjustments to your treatment plan, you can effectively manage BED and work towards sustained recovery. Remember that progress is a journey, and it's okay to seek support and guidance along the way. Be patient, persistent, and proactive in advocating for your health and well-being as you navigate the process of recovery from binge eating disorder.

CELEBRATING SUCCESSES AND STAYING MOTIVATED

Celebrating accomplishments and being motivated are critical components of treating binge eating disorder (BED) and making progress toward recovery. Recognizing and acknowledging your achievements, no matter how small, can boost confidence, reinforce positive behaviors, and provide encouragement to continue on your journey towards healing. Here are some strategies for celebrating successes and staying motivated in the context of BED:

1. **Acknowledge Progress**: Take time to acknowledge and celebrate your progress and achievements, no matter how minor they may seem. Recognize the steps you've taken towards managing BED, whether it's practicing mindful eating, seeking support, or challenging negative thoughts and behaviors.

2. **Set Realistic Goals**: Set realistic, achievable goals for yourself and celebrate each milestone along the way. Break larger goals into smaller, more manageable steps, and celebrate your progress as you work towards accomplishing them.

3. **Practice Gratitude**: Cultivate an attitude of gratitude by focusing on the positive aspects of your life and recovery journey. Express gratitude for the support of friends and family, the progress you've made, and the lessons you've learned along the way.

4. **Reward Yourself**: Treat yourself to rewards or incentives for reaching milestones or achieving goals related to managing BED. Choose rewards that align with your values and promote self-care, such as taking a relaxing bath, indulging in a favorite hobby, or treating yourself to a small gift or activity.

5. **Create a Success Journal**: Keep a success journal or gratitude journal to document your achievements, progress, and moments of gratitude. Write down positive experiences, victories, and moments of pride to reflect on during challenging times.

6. **Celebrate Non-Scale Victories**: Shift your focus away from the number on the scale and celebrate non-scale victories related to managing BED and improving your overall well-being. Celebrate improvements in mood, energy levels, self-esteem, and body image, as well as positive changes in your eating behaviors and coping skills.

7. **Share Your Successes**: Share your successes and achievements with supportive friends, family members, or members of your treatment team. Celebrate your progress with others who understand and validate your experiences, and allow yourself to bask in their encouragement and praise.

8. **Visualize Success**: Visualize yourself achieving your goals and imagine how it will feel to overcome challenges and obstacles along the way. Create a vision board or visualization exercises to reinforce your motivation and commitment to recovery.

9. **Stay Connected to Your Why**: Stay connected to your reasons for wanting to manage

BED and improve your relationship with food and your body. Remind yourself of the benefits of recovery, such as improved health, increased self-esteem, and enhanced quality of life, to stay motivated during difficult times.

10. **Seek Support and Encouragement:** Lean on your support network of friends, family members, or support groups for encouragement, validation, and accountability. Share your successes and challenges with others who can offer empathy, understanding, and motivation to keep going.

By celebrating successes, expressing gratitude, setting realistic goals, and staying connected to your reasons for wanting to manage BED, you can stay motivated and inspired on your journey towards recovery. Remember that progress takes time, patience, and perseverance, and be kind to yourself as you navigate the ups and downs of recovery from binge eating disorder.

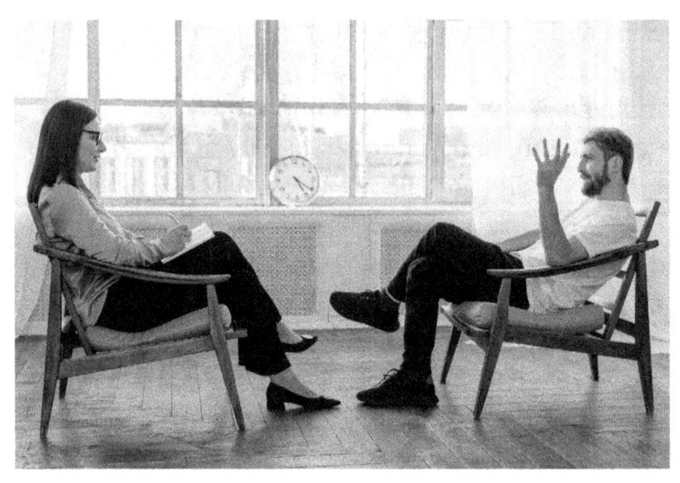

CONCLUSION

In conclusion, managing binge eating disorder (BED) requires a multifaceted approach that addresses underlying factors, builds coping skills, and promotes long-term recovery. Throughout this guide, we have explored various strategies and techniques for understanding, addressing, and overcoming BED. From recognizing triggers and coping mechanisms to seeking professional help and developing a support network, each step plays a vital role in the journey towards healing.

By understanding the complexities of BED and exploring potential underlying causes, individuals can gain insight into their eating behaviors and develop personalized treatment plans. Strategies such as mindfulness, stress management, and balanced meal planning empower individuals to make healthier choices and break free from the cycle of binge eating.

Seeking professional help, whether through therapy, counseling, or support groups, provides essential guidance and support on the path to recovery. By working with trained professionals and building a strong support network, individuals can find validation, encouragement, and accountability in their recovery journey.

Furthermore, practicing self-compassion, celebrating successes, and staying motivated are crucial aspects of maintaining progress and preventing relapse. By acknowledging achievements, expressing gratitude, and staying connected to their reasons for recovery, individuals can stay motivated and inspired on their path towards healing.

In essence, managing binge eating disorder is a journey that requires patience, persistence, and self-awareness. By implementing the strategies outlined in this guide and remaining committed to self-care and self-improvement, individuals can reclaim their relationship with food, cultivate a healthier lifestyle, and experience lasting freedom from binge eating disorder.

RECAP OF KEY POINTS

Here's a recap of the key points discussed in managing binge eating disorder (BED):

1. **Understanding BED**: Recognize the signs and symptoms of BED, including recurrent episodes of binge eating, feelings of loss of control, and distress related to eating behaviors.

2. **Addressing Triggers**: Identify emotional, environmental, and physiological triggers that contribute to binge eating episodes and develop coping strategies to manage them effectively.

3. **Building Coping Skills**: Develop healthy coping mechanisms for managing stress, emotions, and triggers without turning to food, including mindfulness, relaxation techniques, and stress management strategies.

4. **Seeking Professional Help**: Consider seeking support from therapists, counselors, or healthcare providers who specialize in treating BED to explore underlying issues, develop coping strategies, and receive guidance on the recovery journey.

5. **Developing a Support System**: Build a strong support network of friends, family members, or support groups who can offer encouragement, validation, and accountability in managing BED.

6. **Setting Realistic Goals**: Set achievable, behavior-based goals for managing BED and celebrate each milestone along the way to stay motivated and focused on progress.

7. **Monitoring Progress and Making Adjustments**: Regularly assess your progress, track behaviors and symptoms, and make necessary adjustments to your treatment plan to ensure it remains effective and relevant to your needs.

8. **Celebrating Successes**: Acknowledge and celebrate your achievements, no matter how small,

to boost confidence, reinforce positive behaviors, and stay motivated on your recovery journey.

9. **Staying Committed**: Stay committed to your recovery journey, prioritize self-care, and remain patient and persistent in overcoming challenges and obstacles along the way.

10. **Maintaining Long-Term Recovery**: Focus on maintaining progress and preventing relapse by practicing self-care, seeking support, and staying connected to your reasons for wanting to manage BED.

By implementing these key points and strategies, individuals can effectively manage BED, promote long-term recovery, and reclaim their relationship with food and their bodies. Remember that recovery is a journey, and each step forward is a testament to your strength and resilience.

ENCOURAGEMENT FOR CONTINUED PROGRESS AND GROWTH

As you continue on your journey towards managing binge eating disorder and fostering long-term recovery, it's important to remember that progress is not always linear, but every step forward is a testament to your strength, resilience, and determination. Here's some encouragement to support you along the way:

1. **You Are Stronger Than You Know**: Despite the challenges you may face, remember that you possess an inner strength and resilience that will guide you through difficult times. Trust in your ability to overcome obstacles and emerge stronger on the other side.

2. **Celebrate Your Progress**: Take time to acknowledge and celebrate the progress you've made, no matter how small. Each step forward, each victory, and each moment of growth is a testament to your courage and perseverance.

3. **You Deserve Healing and Happiness**: Remind yourself that you are worthy of living a life free from the control of binge eating disorder. Embrace self-compassion and treat yourself with the kindness and understanding you would offer to a loved one facing similar struggles.

4. **Stay Focused on Your Goals**: Keep your goals and aspirations in mind as you navigate the ups and downs of recovery. Stay focused on the positive changes you're working towards and let them guide you forward, even in moments of doubt or uncertainty.

5. **You Are Not Alone**: Remember that you are not alone on this journey. Reach out for support from trusted friends, family members, or

professionals who can offer encouragement, guidance, and understanding along the way.

6. **Every Challenge Is an Opportunity for Growth**: View each challenge or setback as an opportunity for growth and learning. Embrace the lessons that come with overcoming obstacles and use them to propel yourself forward on your path to recovery.

7. **Take One Day at a Time**: Focus on taking things one day at a time and be gentle with yourself as you navigate the complexities of recovery. Embrace the present moment and trust that each step forward brings you closer to healing and wholeness.

8. **Believe in Yourself**: Believe in your ability to overcome adversity, rise above challenges, and create the life you envision for yourself. Cultivate confidence in your resilience and know that you have the power to shape your own destiny.

9. **You Are Worthy of Love and Acceptance**: Remind yourself that your worth is not defined by your struggles or setbacks. You are inherently worthy of love, acceptance, and compassion, regardless of your past experiences or current challenges.

10. **Keep Moving Forward**: No matter how difficult the road may seem, keep moving forward

with courage, determination, and hope. Trust in your ability to navigate the challenges ahead and know that brighter days lie ahead on your journey towards healing and growth.

You've already taken the first steps towards managing binge eating disorder and reclaiming control of your life. Stay committed to your recovery journey, remain open to growth and transformation, and know that you have the strength within you to overcome any obstacle that comes your way.

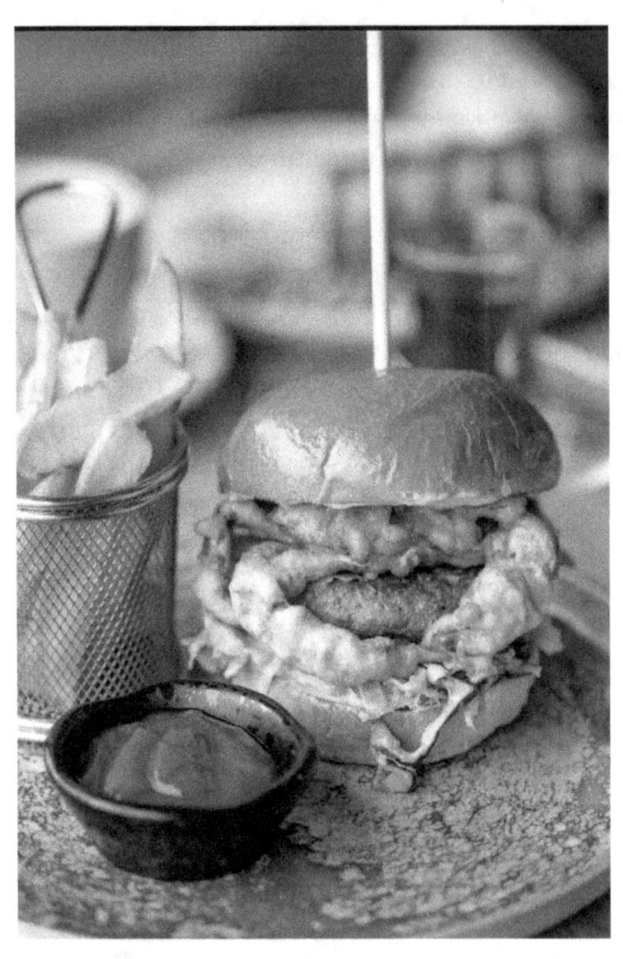

www.ingramcontent.com/pod-product-compliance
Lightning Source LLC
Chambersburg PA
CBHW070806260726
48660CB00005B/1736